From Arsenic to Biologicals:
A 200 Year History of Psoriasis

Barbara S. Baker

G P *Garner Press*

Published by:
Garner Press, PO Box 382, Beckenham, BR3 3UU, UK

From Arsenic to Biologicals: A 200 Year History of Psoriasis
Copyright © 2008 Garner Press

ISBN: 978-0-9551603-2-5

Contents

Preface

Psoriasis is an ancient disease that was probably first described by Hippocrates more than 400 years BC, but was not recognised as a specific clinical entity until the beginning of the 19th century, after more than 600 years of being confused with leprosy.

This book follows, chronologically, the change in the approach to treatment of psoriasis from the "try it and see if it works" to evidence-based therapies driven by an increased understanding of the mechanisms underlying the disease.

Clearly much has been learnt about psoriasis after 200 years of observation, research and treatment, particularly during the latter half of the 20th century. This has been made possible by major technological advances, such as the Human Genome project which facilitated the search for psoriasis genes. It is expected that answers to many of the questions now posed will emerge during the 21st century in association with further technological progress, and, it is hoped, will ultimately lead to the development of a therapy that will switch off the disease permanently.

I hope that both individuals who have psoriasis and professionals who are involved in treating or investigating the disease will find this book of interest.

Many thanks to everybody who has helped me in this venture.

Barbara S. Baker, PhD

~ 1 ~

Recognition of psoriasis as a specific disease

Psoriasis: what's in a name?

Psoriasis is an ancient disease that was probably amongst the scaly eruptions described by Hippocrates (460-377 BC) in his collection of medical dissertations known as the *Hippocratic Corpus*. Hippocrates classified skin conditions into those resulting from "distemper" of the humours (blood, mucous, yellow and black bile) within the body, which included dry scaly eruptions termed lopoi (from *lepo* to scale) such as psoriasis and pityriasis, and those localised to the skin. He also described a skin condition following a sore throat, probably the first description of guttate psoriasis.

The earliest remedies for skin conditions, described in the *Papyrus Ebers* written about 1500 BC, were unsavoury sounding concoctions which included cat and dog's dung for the scurf, and a mixture of onions, sea salt and urine to drive away leprous spots[1]. For scabs, a mixture of fresh oil, goose oil and semen, or wasp's dung in milk of the sycamore was recommended. In addition, "scribe's excrement mixed thoroughly in fresh milk and applied as a poultice" was described as an excellent treatment after scales had been removed.

At the beginning of the first century, psoriasis was described by the Roman scholar Aurelieus Celsus (25 BC–AD 45) in his *De re medica* who referred to it as "impetigo" (from *impeto* meaning attack). He treated the disease with "red nitre and sulfur". Subsequently Galen (AD 133-200) was the first to use the term "psoriasis" (from *psora* meaning to itch), but was probably not referring to psoriasis as we understand it today, but to seborrhoeic eczema. His remedy was broth in which a viper had been boiled, which amazingly was still being recommended as a treatment by Daniel Turner in the 18th century.

In the Bible, psoriasis (and other skin disorders) was considered to be the same as leprosy. The Syrian Naaman the leper who was, we are told, cured of his skin lesions by bathing in the river Jordan, most probably had psoriasis. In the Middle Ages, this confusion between psoriasis and leprosy became more established. True leprosy, known to the Greeks in the

1

2nd century as "elephantiasis graecorum", became confused with "lepra graecorum" when Arabic texts were translated into Latin. The term "lepra" was derived from the Greek *lopos* (epidermis) and *lepo* and included dry scaling conditions such as psoriasis, pityriasis and ichthyosis. Thus there were probably thousands of people suffering from psoriasis who, during the 13th and 14th centuries in Europe, were forced to carry a bell or clapper to warn the healthy population, wore special clothing, and were banned from touching, talking above a whisper, or eating with anyone other than a leper. It has even been suggested by Bechet that, in 1313, Philip the Fair of France ordered individuals with psoriasis to be burnt at the stake[2].

During the Byzantine period, a change in the attitude towards the sick with disfiguring diseases such as leprosy led to them being fed and cared for in monasteries. Some evidence that this included individuals with psoriasis has been recently been unearthed from a monastery in the Judean desert; the skeletal remains of two adult males were found showing characteristic lesions of psoriatic arthritis[3]. A reference to "leprosy" together with deformities of the hands and other joints, including the spine, was later made in a 17th text written by Fray Felipe Columbo describing the life of a monk in Peru called Fray Pedro de Urraca, who was afflicted for more than 29 years with the disease[4].

This inability to distinguish psoriasis from leprosy was to continue for a further five hundred years. For example, numerous references to "leprosy" were found at the middle of the 18th century in the admissions register of the Manchester Infirmary. The description of the skin disease in most of these cases was, however, consistent with a diagnosis of psoriasis[3].

Psoriasis as a clinical entity

The first written work on dermatology describing diseases of the skin was credited to Girolamo Mercuriale in 1572 and was written in Latin. In 1714, Daniel Turner published the first textbook on the subject in the English language (*De morbis cutaneis. A treatise of diseases incident to the skin*), which was, in common with the Mercuriale book, a summary of the literature. This work, which had several editions and was translated into French and German, described all the skin disorders known at the time. Interestingly, Turner separated the skin conditions resembling leprosy and psoriasis into separate chapters suggesting that he may have recognised the two diseases as separate entities. Turner was also the first to use ammoniated mercury ointment as a local treatment for psoriasis,

2

Leper in costume, with clapper and basket. Dictionaire illustre, Paris, 19th century. Wellcome Library, London

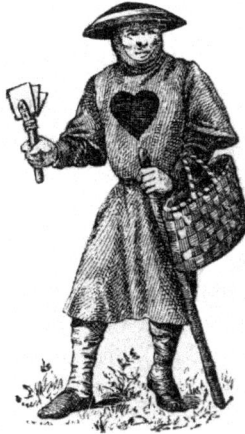

which was still in common use some 200 years later.

More than 60 years later in 1777, a massive text in Latin by the French dermatologist, Anne-Charles Lorry gave the first description of the skin as a living organ. Previously to this, the skin had been regarded as merely a cover for the body. It was a Viennese physician, Joseph Jacob Ritter von Plenck who first attempted, in 1776, to classify skin diseases into categories on the basis of clinical appearance. In his book entitled *Doctrina de morbis cutaneis* (Teachings on the Diseases of the Skin), he arranged the 115 known types of skin diseases into 14 classes. As a result, Plenck is regarded as the founder of the modern classification of skin diseases.

It was not until the beginning of the 19th century that psoriasis was recognised as being a specific clinical entity. This was attributed to Robert Willan, born in 1757 to a Quaker family in Sedbergh, Yorkshire, who was appointed in 1783 as physician to the newly established Carey Street Dispensary in London. In addition to treating outpatients, Willan visited the sick in the slums where infections were rife and the filthy, squalid conditions encouraged a variety of skin conditions. The study of the latter became his life's work and, recognising the value of Plenck's classification, he set out to revise and update it. This led to a new classification system, based upon that used by Linneaus for the animal and plant kingdoms. Willan defined, in detail, 10 (later 12) morphological types of skin lesions using terms such as scale, papula and pustule that we are familiar with today. From these lesion types, he divided skin diseases into eight Orders according to their clinical appearance, which he defined precisely and in great detail.

The first four Orders were published in 1808 in a book entitled *On Cutaneous Diseases*. This was the first textbook of skin diseases to be systematically illustrated, containing 34 copper-engraved, hand coloured plates showing the characteristic morphological appearances of the different skin conditions. In addition to recognising psoriasis as a specific clinical entity in this treatise, Willan was the first to describe its different clinical forms. He also revived the term "psoriasis" which hadn't been used since Galen's inappropriate use of it more than 1600 years previously, naming the serpiginous (spreading) form of psoriasis as "psoriasis gyrata". However, he was unable to separate psoriasis from leprosy completely and continued to refer to the more common form of psoriasis (chronic plaque) as "lepra vulgaris".

Willan became ill and died in Madeira in April 1812 at the age of 55 years, before being able to complete the second volume that was to contain the remaining four of his Orders. His pupil and friend, Thomas Bateman, who succeeded him as physician at the Carey Street Dispensary in 1804, took up the task of completing the classification of skin diseases. He bought the copyright of Willan's work and of the watercolour drawings that accompanied it and subsequently published his own work entitled *A Practical Synopsis on Cutaneous Diseases* in 1813. Several editions of this work were published and it was translated into five foreign languages. So successful was the book that the Emperor of Russia ordered several copies and even presented Bateman with a ring worth 100 guineas to show his admiration!

Thus Willan and Bateman precisely defined the descriptive terms used and assigned individual diseases into a single class, thus avoiding the separation of different stages of the same disease into different classes, which had been a feature of previous attempts at disease classification. This logical approach to disease identification based upon the anatomy of the "elementary" lesion was easy to teach and became widely practiced.

In France, dermatology was established as a speciality at the Hôpital Saint-

Louis, Paris at the end of 1801 when the hospital was officially designated as a centre for chronic skin diseases. Jean-Louis Alibert (1768-1837) was appointed its head and founded the French School of Dermatology. In 1806 he published a tome describing the diseases of the skin (*Description des maladies de la peau*) that was impressive, not least for its hand coloured copperplate engravings, which were of superior quality compared to those of Willan and Bateman. Alibert's approach to the classification of skin diseases was different to that of Willan and Bateman and encompassed several criteria such as cause, course, duration, appearance and response to treatment. The result was a somewhat confusing system of classification, famously represented by his "tree of dermatoses" which was first published in 1832. Alibert's system of classification was, however, generally discarded after his pupil, the Swiss-born Laurent-Theodore Biett, was introduced to the Willan-Bateman method of clinical diagnosis on a visit to the Carey Street Dispensary. When these concepts were presented in France in 1816, most French dermatologists enthusiastically adopted them.

Subsequently, dermatology as a speciality was also established in the United States. Henry Daggett Bulkley, who trained under Biett (and Cazenave) in Paris in 1831, opened the Broome Street Dispensary in New York in 1836 and thus established the first institution in the United States for the treatment of skin diseases.

In the 1840s, a new era of dermatology began with the work of Ferdinand von Hebra who founded the first German school of Dermatology in Vienna. He published a new classification of skin diseases based upon the pathological anatomy of the skin. This new system replaced all the previous methods of classification and laid the foundation for a new science. Hebra is therefore regarded as the founder of modern dermatology, and in 1849 was the first dermatologist to be appointed specifically as a professor of skin diseases. Under Hebra's direction, Vienna in the 1860s became the international centre for dermatological training and research. In addition, it was Hebra that finally eliminated the word "lepra" from the clinical description of psoriasis, thus bringing to an end the confusion between leprosy and psoriasis that had reigned for centuries.

~ 2 ~

Causes and treatments of psoriasis in the 19th Century

A disease of the internal organs or skin?

At the beginning of the 19th century, it was already accepted that psoriasis was an inherited disease. Possible causes that were favoured included stomach and bowel disorders, a functional weakness of nerves in the skin, and mental disease; an association with syphilis was also implicated. In addition, several other factors were believed to worsen the disease, including the consumption of certain foods such as dried meats, fish or oatmeal, violent exercise and cold water, contact with powdery substances (bakers, bricklayers, coal men and dust men) and a lack of personal hygiene. Generally it was believed that psoriasis was the result of an internal disturbance rather than a local defect of the skin.

In the middle of the 19th century in Vienna, Hebra recognised the need to determine the pathological processes involved in the development of the disease, and so proceeded to carry out post-mortems on patients with psoriasis who had died from other complaints[1]. He concluded that psoriasis did not arise as a result of internal organ disease, as generally believed, but was initiated externally. Furthermore, his examination of 3,000 cases of psoriasis per year showed that individuals with psoriasis were of strong constitution, well nourished and with normal bodily functions. He dismissed the suggestions made by other dermatologists that uncleanliness, the seasons, geographical location, contagion or cold temperatures were causative of psoriasis, but proposed the idea that any irritant applied to the skin may cause an eruption of psoriatic lesions in predisposed individuals. An observation reported by Heinrich Koebner in 1877 provided evidence for this proposed role of external factors in the initiation of psoriasis[2]. He described the appearance of psoriatic lesions in the normal-looking skin of psoriatic patients at sites of trauma such as tattoos, abrasions and horse bites. This was subsequently referred to as the Koebner reaction or phenomenon, when induced experimentally.

A possible role for infections in psoriasis was also being considered at this time. In 1878, Lang[3] suggested that psoriasis was a parasitic affection caused by an "epidermidophyton" present in psoriatic scales. This alleged fungus was also found by other workers, but was subsequently shown by Ries[4] to be an artifact caused by the presence of minute granules of débris within the cell cytoplasm (termed eleidin). The presence in psoriatic skin of micrococci, "bottle" bacilli (probably the yeast *Pityrosporum ovale*), or minute circular bodies with dark central spots arranged in loose clusters or dense masses were also reported. Even cases of alleged transmission to other unrelated individuals were recorded.

Further suggestive evidence for a causative role for micro-organisms in psoriasis came from the observation that skin lesions could be induced by vaccination, a procedure that was to become widely practised after Pasteur's demonstration of induction of immunity to cholera in chickens in 1880. In one study in 1882, itchy, scaly skin lesions appeared at the site of inoculation in two psoriasis patients, 8 or 9 days after vaccination with fresh bovine virus, which subsequently spread to the arms and legs[5]. Further occasional incidences of vaccination-induced eruptions were also reported.

Histopathology

The first microscopical studies of psoriatic skin lesions were performed in the middle of the 19th century when acromatic microscopes with reduced optical defects became available. These studies revealed that psoriasis consisted of piles of epidermal cells above the corium (dermis) with an increased blood supply. Although no staining of skin tissue was possible at this time, these studies were the first to show that psoriasis was the result of excessive growth of the epidermis. With further technical developments in the latter half of the century, such as better microscopes and the introduction of embedding and staining techniques, detailed histological examinations of psoriatic skin lesions became possible.

Thus all the presently known histological features of the disease were identified by W Allan Jamieson in 1879, including enlarged blood capillaries, infiltrating leukocytes (white cells), formation of epidermal projections or rete ridges, and the presence of nuclei in the top layer of the epidermis (stratum corneum), known as parakeratosis[6]. Jamieson also examined normal-looking skin from the same patients and found it to be similar in appearance to skin from non-psoriatic individuals. On the basis of his observations, he proposed that the first step in the disease process was by the cells of the rete Malpighi (epidermal cells in the rete ridges)

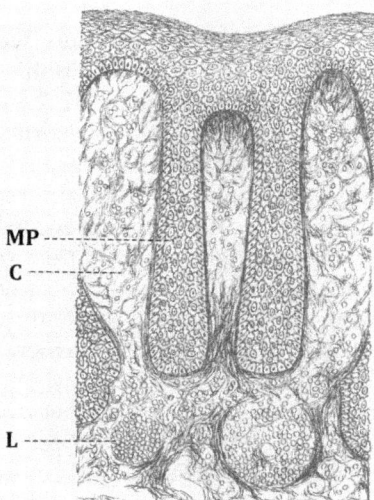

*Histology of a psoriatic skin lesion. From Jamieson WA, Edinburgh Med. J.
1879; 24(7): 622-29. Wellcome Library. London
MP, Malpighian prolongations; C, Corium; L, Leukocytes*

next to the dermis, and not by the dermal papillae, and that this occurred before changes in the blood vessels and infiltration of white cells.

This was one of several different hypotheses that were to be proposed during this and the following century. For example, a further histological study carried out on early skin lesions some 20 years later by Munro[7] concluded that the first changes in the psoriatic process began at the surface of the skin in the stratum corneum. This was based upon his observations of collections of bacteria-engulfing white cells (neutrophils) on the surface of the keratin layer, which he described as being similar to an abscess, later termed "Munro's abscess". Formation of this abscess was considered to be the primary event as neutrophils were observed migrating through the epidermis to a normal-looking keratin layer. Thickening of the keratin layer was postulated to occur under the tiny abscess, which would then be pushed upwards resulting in death of the leukocytes. This would explain the presence of nuclei in the keratin layer. These observations prompted Munro to search for microbes in the skin lesions, but none were detected.

Epidemiology and natural history of the disease

In London, 719 of 10,000 (7.19%) skin patients were diagnosed with psoriasis, as reported by Radcliffe Crocker in his textbook of 1888. This was approximately twice the figure of 2.8–4.2% observed by dermatologists in America and Vienna. Since psoriasis was not difficult to diagnose, (although there were cases that were wrongly diagnosed as syphilis at the beginning of the century), this difference may have been due to individuals with recurrent attacks being recorded more than once. Furthermore, L. Duncan Bulkley observed that the frequency of psoriasis varied in different American cities, being more prevalent in New York (4.1%), Boston and Chicago where there was plenty of rain and marked changes in temperature, and less so in the warmer, drier cities such as Baltimore (1.8%) and St Louis in the south.

In a clinical study and analysis of 1,000 cases of psoriasis seen in New York[8], Bulkley made various, mostly accurate, observations on the clinical characteristics of the disease. He noted that slightly more males (53.1%) than females were affected, that the disease tended to appear most frequently at around 20-25 years and relatively rarely in the first few years of life, and that the disease was chronic, lasting years with no tendency for self-limitation. Although it was generally accepted at the time that there was a hereditary element to psoriasis, Bulkley considered that this played only a small part in the onset of the disease. This was based upon his analysis of 385 psoriatic individuals of which only 33 had parents or grandparents who also had the disease. In addition, he noted that approximately 10% of children of psoriatic individuals and 14% of their siblings were psoriatic.

Recognised external triggers of skin lesions at the time were pregnancy and lactation, vaccination, scarlatina, acute dermal inflammation, fear, grief, anxiety, diet and hygiene. An association between psoriasis and rheumatism/gout was also well recognised, particularly by the French school of dermatologists. Bulkley subsequently investigated the urine of psoriatic patients and found a raised specific gravity and hyperacidity that he associated with burning and itching of the skin[9]. He concluded that an "acid blood state" was responsible for both the skin lesions and rheumatism/gout, a hypothesis that failed to survive the test of time!

Treatments

Treatments for psoriasis in the 19th century were given empirically since their mode of action was unknown. If a treatment appeared to be beneficial, the findings were reported in medical journals such as The Lancet, and its use recommended to other dermatologists. Sometimes comparisons between two local treatments were made after application to separate sites on an individual patient, but there were no formal clinical trials at this time to establish the safety or efficacy of the therapies used. This practice of "try it and see if it works" was to continue until well into the next century and only changed when more became known about the pathogenic mechanisms involved in the psoriatic process.

As mentioned above, current thinking regarded psoriasis as a local manifestation of abnormal internal bodily functions and, as such, required both local and/or internal treatments. Furthermore it was generally believed, in the early part of the century, that the rapid clearance of a skin eruption would result in the "driving in" of the defect. This belief probably stemmed from the observation that skin rashes can disappear in seriously ill patients, mistaking the result for the cause. Internal treatments were more commonly used in England, whilst doctors in Vienna favoured local treatments. However, a combination of both forms of therapy was usually prescribed since complete resolution of the disease was rarely achieved with either approach alone.

Early treatment of psoriasis was believed to be the key to successful resolution of lesions, and it was felt that the longer the disease was left, the more the skin would take on a "bad tendency" which was difficult to normalise. Furthermore, the ability to "cure" the disease was dependent upon factors such as age of disease onset, time of initiation of treatment in relation to disease onset, type of treatment and patient compliance. (Although the word "cure" was often used at this time, it was not meant to imply that the disease would not return on cessation of treatment, as this was well recognised to occur, but merely that complete healing of lesions had been achieved).

Systemic Treatments

At the beginning of the century, bleeding and the use of purgatives and diuretics were still commonly used to treat psoriasis, but these approaches gradually went out of general use and were replaced by a variety of different remedies. The main systemic treatments employed were arsenic, alkaline salts, mercury, pitch, carbolic acid, phosphorus, chrysarobin, thyroid extract and salicin/salicylates (Table).

Table. 19th century treatments for psoriasis

Systemic	Topical
Arsenic: *Fowler's solution, Asiatic pill,* *bread pill*	Soothing: Baths, hydropathic treatment, ointments (e.g. zinc, mercury)
Mercury Alkaline Remedies: *Potassium nitrate* *Potassium acetate* *Nitrous ether*	Stimulating: Tars and their derivatives (wood-tar, coal-tar, oil of Cade, Oleum Rusci, pitch, creosote)
Pitch Chrysarobin Carbolic acid Phosphorus Thyroid extract Salicin/salicylates	Chrysarobin Carbolic acid Pyrogallic acid Turpentine Occlusive therapy (india rubber films and dressings)
Salts: *Magnesium sulphate* *Sodium carbonate* *Rochelle salts*	
Plain diet without rich fatty foods and alcohol	
Spa treatment	

Arsenic

The systemic treatment of choice for psoriasis at this time was arsenic. Arsenic was first mentioned as one of the ingredients of a paste used to treat skin disorders by Hippocrates. In the 18th century, arsenic was sold in England as "tasteless ague drops" or "Edward's ague tincture". Subsequently, Thomas Fowler (1736-1801), an English physician who had previously been an apothecary, developed a formulation of potassium

LIQUOR ARSENICALIS
ARSENICAL SOLUTION

Take of prepared Oxyd of Arsenic in very
fine powder,
Subcarbonate of Potass from Tar-
tar, of each sixty-four grains,
Distilled Water, a pint

Boil them together in a glass vessel until
the arsenic is entirely dissolved. When the
solution is cold, add thereto,

Compound Spirit of Lavender, four
fluid drachms

Lastly add as much more distilled water
as may be requisite to make up a pint measure

Recipe for "Liquor Arsenicalis" or Fowler's Solution

arsenite (known as Fowler's solution) to which he added compound tincture of lavender to give it colour and taste . Girdlestone was the first to use this solution at the beginning of the 19th century to treat psoriasis and other skin diseases such as lepra, lichen and prurigo[10]. Arsenic, which was first introduced into the Pharmacopoeia of the Royal College of Physicians of London in 1809, was subsequently administered in various liquid or pill forms, mixed with substances such as liquor potassae, bicarbonate of soda, iron, breadcrumbs or pepper (Asiatic pill), given three times a day. The doses of arsenic given were usually small, and often had little beneficial effect. Both exacerbation of skin lesions after starting the treatment, and side-effects such as conjunctivitis, gastrointestinal upsets and tingling of the extremities were not uncommon amongst psoriasis patients treated by this regime, although the latter were misconstrued as being indicative of efficacy! Investigation of the effects of arsenic on skin in frogs by Ringer

13

and Murrel revealed that it attacked the columnar epidermal cells next to the blood vessels in the dermis resulting in the eventual removal of the epidermis. It was therefore suggested that this might be its mode of action in psoriasis.

In order to increase the efficacy of arsenic in psoriasis, Shapter, in a report in the Lancet in 1878[11], argued for the administration of higher doses of the drug to patients who had not responded to the usual lines of treatment. He described how giving increasing doses of one twentieth to one half a grain of arsenious acid in a bread pill to 5 cases of psoriasis resulted in almost complete clearing of their skin, and was apparently well tolerated. Today, the idea that a poison such as arsenic should be used as a treatment for psoriasis at doses such as these would be very controversial. Indeed, the smallest recorded fatal dose of arsenic at the time was two grains, only 4 times the highest dose given to one of the 5 patients in the study.

Alkaline treatments

Since arsenic was not an effective therapy at lower doses and many patients were unable to tolerate its side effects, various other remedies were also tried. Alkaline substances such as nitrate of potash (potassium nitrate), acetate of potash (potassium acetate) or nitrous ether, or alternatively, pitch, a tar distillation product, or carbolic acid (see below) in capsule or pill form was sometimes used. These latter medications were believed to act beneficially by stimulating kidney function, thus relieving the skin. Furthermore, psoriasis patients with a "gouty predisposition", (possibly with psoriatic arthritis) were treated with alkaline remedies, occasional use of mercurial purgatives, and sulphates of magnesia and soda (sodium carbonate) or Rochelle salts to "promote more free and watery evacuations from the liver and bowels"[12].

Phosphorus

Phosphorus, first employed in the treatment of psoriasis at the Hôpital Saint-Louis in Paris, was another alternative internal treatment to arsenic in use at this time. This was considered to be a powerful nervine tonic being more potent than carbolic acid, which was in turn more potent than arsenious acid at the respective doses usually administered. However, both phosphorus and carbolic acid caused marked physiological effects in some patients, which necessitated cessation of the treatment before skin lesions had cleared.

Chrysarobin

Chrysarobin (chrysophanic acid) has also been administered internally to treat psoriasis. Chrysarobin is a mixture of substances obtained from araroba, a substance found in the trunk of the Andira Araroba, a large tree growing in the forests of Brazil. However, beneficial effects were variable and slow due to the necessity of using small doses to avoid gastro-intestinal irritation. Chrysarobin is more commonly used as a local treatment, although, even under these circumstances, it appears to be absorbed into the circulation (see below).

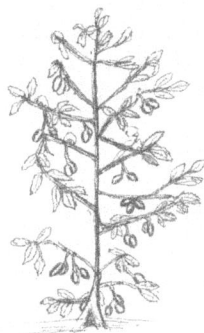

Andira Araroba
Illustration by Betty Baker

At the end of the century, two novel systemic approaches to the treatment of psoriasis were introduced; thyroid extract and salicin/salicylates.

Thyroid extracts

Sir Byrom Bramwell, a Scottish physician, proposed the use of thyroid extract in psoriasis patients, based upon the observation that patients with cretinism had a marked improvement in the quality of their skin after being fed with thyroid glands. The findings of a case series of 20 psoriasis patients with varying degrees of disease activity, who were treated by Bramwell with either minced raw gland wrapped in rice paper, or extract, dried or liquid, were reported in his "Atlas of Clinical Medicine"[13]. Thirteen patients who had received the higher doses of thyroid extract for an average of 3 months responded to the treatment, but their disease relapsed after 1 year. Despite some other reports attesting to the resolution of psoriasis in response to treatment with thyroid extract, these findings were not generally reproduced and so-called "thyroid feeding" went out of favour. Interestingly, recent evidence has been found for a link between thyroid gland dysfunction and palmaplantar psoriasis, suggesting that Bramwell's hypothesis that patients with psoriasis may be deficient in endogenous thyroid secretion may have been correct after all, at least in certain subtypes of the disease.

15

Salicin/Salicylates

Salicin/salicylates, obtained from the bark of the Salix (willow) and Populus (poplar) trees, had proved beneficial in diseases such as rheumatism. On this basis, they were recommended by Radcliffe Crocker for use in psoriasis [14]. He reported the success of this treatment particularly in patients with acute guttate psoriasis of short duration, for whom thyroid extract, which exacerbated the disease, and arsenic were generally found to be unsuitable. However, a less striking beneficial effect of the drugs was found in patients with only a few chronic patches. The treatment was not found generally to aggravate the disease, but did cause dyspepsia in some patients soon after it was taken. It was suggested that salicylates may resolve psoriasis by acting as anti-microbial agents in the blood. Indeed, it was believed that carbolic acid, mercury and arsenic also acted as microbicides. As we now know, salicylic acid (aspirin) is a non-steroidal anti-inflammatory drug, which is consistent with the pale appearance of the treated skin lesions observed by Radcliffe Crocker.

For many patients, these remedies must have been very hard to stomach (literally!) with their attendant unpleasant side-effects and slow, or non-existent beneficial effects. Some of these substances were also applied locally (pitch, carbolic acid, chrysarobin; see below), sometimes with adverse constitutional consequences as a result of absorption through the skin. A visit to a spa was believed to be helpful as an accompaniment to treatment, and a plain diet, avoiding rich fatty foods, animal meat, wines and malt liquors, and the drinking of plenty of water was recommended. It seems that the stimulatory effects of alcohol on psoriasis have been recognised for more than 100 years.

Topical treatments

The choice of topical treatments used in the 19th century for inflammatory skin conditions was dependent upon whether the eruption was considered acute or chronic. Thus soothing treatments were applied in the acute cases, whilst chronic skin conditions were subjected to more stimulating applications (Table).

16

Baths, ointments or lotions

Soothing treatments included baths, ointments or lotions. In acute psoriasis covering a large extent of the body, warm baths to which washing soda, glycerine or starch was added were recommended. Hydropathic treatment was also used, especially in those cases where the skin was hot and itchy. This involved placing the naked patient on a cold, wet sheet and wrapping it tightly around him/her so that all the skin was covered, and then covering with a blanket and tying it into place with straps. The patient would then remain in this state for approximately 3 hours, being encouraged to drink plenty of water to encourage sweating. After removal of the wrappings, the patient was plunged into a cold bath and the skin rubbed before and after drying. A brisk walk finished off the procedure. It is difficult to imagine that this treatment could be considered soothing!

Ointments were used to soften and facilitate the removal of scales, but predominately to protect the affected skin from the air. They contained a variety of substances such as benzoated oxide of zinc, nitric oxide of mercury and calomel (mercurous chloride).

In cases of chronic psoriasis, the scales were removed from the lesional skin before applying any local treatment to aid healing. This was often achieved using potash applications such as potash soap, liquor potassae or solutions of potassa fusa, or by rubbing in olive oil for one week and covering in bandages soaked in olive oil. The local treatments employed included tars and their derivatives, chrysarobin, carbolic acid, pyrogallic acid, turpentine and prolonged occlusive therapy.

Tars and their derivatives

Tars and their derivatives (wood-tar, coal-tar, oil of Cade, Oleum Rusci, pitch and creosote) were widely used to treat psoriasis and were thought to be good for relieving itching. These could either be applied directly to descaled skin with a brush, or as a component of lotions or ointments in order to reduce their irritant effects. In addition to their ability to irritate the skin, the other main disadvantages to the use of these tarry preparations were their messiness and pungent smell. Although the oil of Cade (extracted from juniper trees) and Oleum Rusci (extracted from the bark of the white birch) were less odious than the others, their higher cost limited their use. The successful use of these ointments required the patient to stay in bed or wear clothes covered in the tarry substances,

17

which must have been extremely uncomfortable. Furthermore, the side-effects experienced whilst using these preparations included black vomit, faeces and urine, shivering, headaches and acne. Treatment with tars was sometimes alternated with the application of mercurial preparations to reduce the side-effects produced by both types of treatments. In 1866, William Valentine Wright created an antiseptic soap from "liquor carbonis detergens", the liquid by-product of the distillation of coal to coke, for the treatment of skin disorders. Wright's coal tar soap was used for over 130 years, but succumbed to an European Union directive to remove coal tar from non-prescription products. However, coal tar extract is still used today in shampoos for the treatment of scalp psoriasis, a testament to its effectiveness in the regulation of skin cell proliferation.

Chrysarobin

Chrysarobin, although occasionally given internally as a treatment for psoriasis (see above), was more commonly used as an ointment because of its irritant effects on the digestive system. However, there was evidence that, when applied topically to the skin, the drug was absorbed, sometimes inducing nausea, vomiting and diarrhoea, and resulting in the healing of lesions on untreated areas. The ointment required careful use as it caused conjunctivitis, burning of the skin if insufficiently diluted, and staining of both skin and clothes. Furthermore, it could not be used for the scalp as it stained the hair a purple colour.

Not unusually in the history of psoriasis treatment, the usefulness of chrysarobin was found by accident when a patient from Hong Kong with annular psoriatic lesions was mistakenly thought to have a ringworm infection and was treated with an Indian remedy, Goa powder, which contained the substance as its main ingredient. The anti-parasitic effects of the drug and its beneficial effects in psoriasis thus lent support to Lang's parasitic hypothesis for the disease. In common with coal tar, this is one of the few treatments employed in the 19th century that it is still in use today, although in its synthetic form anthralin (dithranol). However, its mode of action in psoriasis is still only partially understood.

Carbolic acid

The use of carbolic acid (phenol) to treat psoriasis was first reported by Dr John McNab who, writing in the Lancet in 1870[15], proposed that psoriasis consisted of a generic inflammation of unknown cause which induced morbid secretions that took the form of scaly encrustations; a hypothesis not unsimilar to those espoused today. Further, McNab proposed that, even when the inflammation abated, the altered function of the skin would remain unless corrected by appropriate local remedies. This prediction is supported by current genetic studies which show defects of epidermal genes that may contribute to the disease process.

Based upon this theory, and the then recently published observations by Lister of the antiseptic treatment of wounds, McNab began to treat a patient with resistant psoriasis with carbolic acid in ointment form (mixed 1:4 with common lard, melted down, mixed and then allowed to cool). After continuing the treatment for some time, the scales began to fall off, epidermal growth slowed down and the skin began to look more normal. At this point the carbolic acid was replaced by oxide-of-zinc ointment for a short period until the lesions disappeared completely. McNab also treated further treatment-resistant patients with some success by combining topical carbolic acid with liquor arsenicalis and other systemic agents used to combat the general predisposition to the disease.

To explain the beneficial effects of carbolic acid in psoriasis, McNab suggested, firstly, that it acted chemically on the organic compounds in the skin resulting in coagulation of the exudate that he had hypothesized mediated the skin changes. Secondly, he suggested that carbolic acid neutralised any local effects exerted by oxygen in the air on the skin. With hindsight, it is likely that the therapeutic effects were partly explained by the fact that the carbolic acid was applied under occlusion to prevent evaporation, a method of application which has been recently shown to act alone, or in synergy with effective treatments, to clear psoriatic skin lesions. Furthermore, the anti-microbial effects of carbolic acid may have also contributed to the resolution of the skin lesions.

Pyrogallic acid

Another phenolic compound, pyrogallic acid, has also been applied in ointment form to skin lesions of psoriasis with some success[16]. It produced a faster and more complete healing of the skin as compared to white precipitate ointment or oil of Cade, and, despite acting as an irritant when used at high concentrations, it did not cause the side-effects associated with the use of chrysarobin. However, when pyrogallic acid was used to treat a large surface area in patients with extensive psoriasis, absorption of the substance led to systemic symptoms of moderate fever and malaise, and dark-coloured urine. Furthermore, in one case, the effects of the treatment were so severe that rigors, coma and subsequently death resulted.

Turpentine

Another remedy sometimes used to treat chronic psoriasis was turpentine suspended in an emulsion, which was apparently as effective as chrysarobin. Although it was a much cleaner substance to apply than the latter, its smell gave it a distinct disadvantage.

India Rubber

A different approach to the local treatment of chronic psoriasis was that of covering the skin to prevent evaporation. This was achieved using india rubber, either in the form of a solution that formed a film over the skin or by the use of dressings.

A solution of india rubber (or gutta-percha, sap from the Malayan Isonandra tree) in chloroform was applied thickly with a brush to skin that had been descaled and wiped free of grease. This application was renewed as often as necessary in order to maintain a continuous covering over the affected skin. After about 3 weeks, the skin became supple and any scales were removed together with the covering leaving a red mark that gradually faded. A modification of this approach was the addition of chrysarobin to a gutta-percha solution; this produced a more rapid response without the problem of staining.

Prolonged occlusive therapy

Prolonged occlusive therapy was used to treat psoriasis during the latter half of the 19th century in Vienna, particularly by Hebra, but was not popular in England or the United States where systemic treatments were generally favoured over topical remedies. The treatment involved the use of india-rubber dressings, which became available after the development of the rubber vulcanisation process by Charles Goodyear in 1839. The flexible rubber cloth was used to make gloves, stockings, caps, bandages and even a complete set of underclothing. It can only be imagined how uncomfortable it must have been to walk around all day sweating underneath these rubber clothes! The rubber was thought to act by excluding the air, keeping the skin warm and at a uniform temperature, and by promoting sweat secretion, which it retained, facilitating the maceration and removal of the epidermis. Sulphur present in the rubber was also thought to be a possible contributory factor. At the end of the century its use was discontinued, partly because of the problem of patient compliance, and partly because of the serious cases of acute dermatitis (later classified as allergic contact dermatitis) that arose from its use.

Thus the 19th century began with the belief that psoriasis resulted from a defect of the internal organs requiring the traditional methods of treatment, such as bleeding and purging. This view gradually changed as the century progressed and more became known about the natural history of the disease and the cellular nature of the skin lesions. A variety of different substances were tested, empirically, for their ability to inhibit the disease process, and scientific explanations for how these treatments worked were sought. By the end of the century, external treatments became more important as a means of resolving psoriasis, but their side-effects were many, their efficacy variable and their mode of action was largely unknown.

~ 3 ~

1900 - 1930

Two main theories for the cause of psoriasis had been proposed during the 19th century; metabolic (endocrine or neuropathic) and parasitic. As the new century began, opinions began to change and the microbial theory began to gain new ground as more observations of the presence of microorganisms in psoriatic skin were published. In addition, a new hypothesis proposing a primary defect of the epidermis was published.

Advances in technology throughout the 20th century were to play a major role in the development of more effective therapies for psoriasis. This process began early on in the century when new discoveries in the field of physics led to the use of radiation therapy in psoriasis.

A microbial aetiology?

Bacteria and/or yeast were reported in skin lesions of psoriasis in various studies. lending support to a microbial cause for the disease. In 1910, Serrell Cooke carried out a bacteriological study of active skin lesions from 20 patients with psoriasis at St John's Hospital in London[1]. He isolated bacteria resembling *Staphylococcus aureus*, and yeast, from many of the lesions, and also a short stumpy Gram-positive bacillus that had not previously been described in association with psoriasis. Further evidence for the presence of a bacillus in psoriatic skin lesions was reported approximately 25 years later (see Chapter 4), but has not been confirmed in contemporary studies.

The possible role of monilia in psoriasis was investigated in detail by a group of American dermatologists[2]. Monilia, meaning "necklace", is a yeast mainly represented by *Candida albicans* which is responsible for thrush and associated infections. Monilia was demonstrated in the skin lesions of just over a third of 56 psoriasis patients (and in the blood of a few patients). This was different from the skin of patients with various forms of eczema, in which the yeast was observed only infrequently. In normal skin, monilia appeared to be totally absent. Additionally, monilia was recovered from the stools of a large number of the psoriasis patients, compared to only a few of the controls or patients with gastrointestinal

23

complaints. Psoriasis patients were also more likely than controls to show a strong skin response to the yeast. This was tested by applying a few drops of an emulsion of killed yeast to abraded skin.

A possible therapeutic effect of vaccination with killed cultured monilia was also investigated as part of the study, but was only partially successful. Lesions reappeared in some cases shortly after treatment was discontinued, and even, in a few, during administration of the vaccine suggesting that the effects were non-specific.

Although the increased presence and response to monilia was consistent with a role for the organism in psoriasis, attempts to induce psoriasis in (animals or) patients were unsuccessful, suggesting that a causal relationship between monilia and the disease was lacking.

Strickler and Asnis[3] reported increased circulating numbers of lymphocytes (lymphocytosis) in half of a group of 27 patients with psoriasis of varying type, severity and extent, and argued that this supported the proposed role of bacteria in psoriasis. This was based upon the fact that marked lymphocytosis is often found in chronic infectious diseases such as tuberculosis.

Although the above findings were suggestive of a microbial aetiology for psoriasis, the presence of microorganisms on lesional skin were also interpreted by some at the time as a secondary phenomenon resulting from the "relatively poor reactive powers" of the psoriatic lesion. In fact, we now know that there are high levels of anti-microbial factors in psoriatic skin which can kill bacteria, and that skin infections are rare. Furthermore, a report of six cases of psoriasis following tonsillitis[4] introduced the possibility that bacteria may indeed be responsible for triggering the disease, but from a different site in the body, more evidence for which was to emerge later.

A primary defect of the skin?

In contrast to the microbial theory for psoriasis, a new hypothesis by Samberger[5] proposed that the true cause of the disease was a congenital, sometimes hereditary defect of the keratin-forming cells. This defect was suggested by the observation that psoriatics (in his experience) do not normally produce a corn in response to trauma caused by manual labour or an ill-fitting boot. This was interpreted as a failure of the corneous layer to increase in size in the normal way resulting in the formation of scaly patches in response to stimuli. Samberger went on to argue that the degree that this skin defect is manifested varies in different individuals, so that the skin of some are easily triggered, whilst others require an external factor, such as a coincident tuberculosis infection or gout, to induce formation of lesions. Furthermore, he believed that the presence of microorganisms on the skin surface was secondary to the inherently defective epidermis, rather than a primary cause of the disease. He suggested that the typical location of the skin lesions (scalp, knees and elbows) supported rather than argued against the theory, because the scalp is a microbial reservoir and the knees and elbows are regions continually exposed to trauma. He even foresaw the possibility of prophylactic treatment for psoriasis in utero, a concept well advance of its time as gene therapy would not start to become a reality for at least another 60 years. Samberger did not, however, exclude the possibility that the abnormality of the skin could be a secondary phenomenon, as a concession to the general belief at that time that psoriasis resulted from an endocrine deficiency.

The idea that skin cells in psoriasis have a genetic alteration which leads to an abnormal response to stimuli and uncontrolled growth is one that has general support by dermatologists today. However, we now know that this is only one of the defects that is required for the disease to be manifested (more about that later).

Treatment

At the turn of the century, Fowler's solution (potassium arsenite) was still being used as a systemic treatment for psoriasis, despite its side effects and variable therapeutic effects. Furthermore, agents such as chrysarobin (in its synthetic form, anthralin) and coal tar remained important topical treatment options , and continued to be so for the next 100 years! However, discoveries made at the beginning of the new century led to the novel use of X-rays, radium and grenz rays to treat psoriasis. In addition, the recognition that ultra violet (UV) rays were responsible for the therapeutic effects of sunlight, and the development of artificial UV lamps resulted in the use of phototherapy in psoriasis.

X- rays and gamma rays

At the beginning of the 20th century, new discoveries in the field of physics began to have a far-reaching impact on medicine. Thus the discovery of X-rays (roentgen rays) by Wilhelm Roentgen in 1895 provided, not only a new diagnostic tool, but a novel approach to the treatment of diseases, including skin diseases such as psoriasis. The observation that prolonged exposure to X-rays induced erythema of the skin, and sometimes dermatitis or even deep ulceration, led to its use as a treatment, initially for nevus, hypertrichosis, cancer and tuberculosis. The first treatment of psoriasis with X-rays was made by Sträter in 1900, and was subsequently used by various dermatologists in England and America, including Dr William Allen Pusey who believed that it was "the most important, single therapeutic agent in the armamentarium of dermatology". Psoriatic skin lesions were found to be sensitive to the effects of X-rays and would disappear quickly with small doses. Small, long-standing lesions resolved

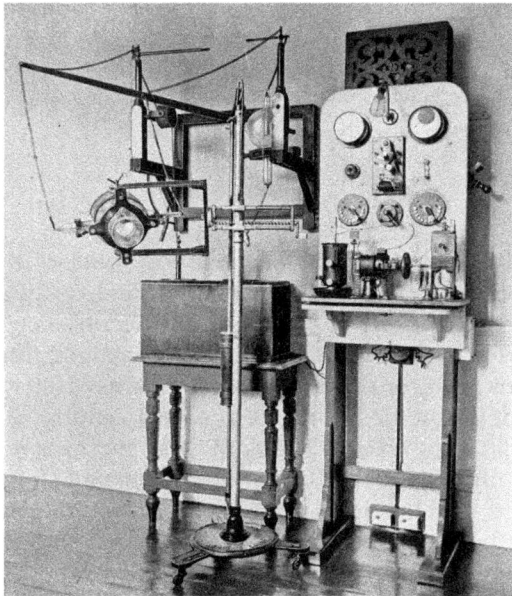

X-ray Apparatus. From "Diseases of the skin" by JMH Macleod, 1920. Wellcome Library, London

after a single semi-intensive or sub-intensive dose, whilst larger, refractive lesions, and generalized eruptions, required 3-8 fractional treatments[6]. Although irradiation did not always clear lesions entirely, improvement was usually obtained. The effectiveness of X-rays in psoriasis was thought to be due to the increased blood supply in the lesions, although previous treatments with agents such as chrysarobin may have contributed to their reactivity. Indeed, such treatment was contra-indicated during X-ray and radium (see below) therapy.

In a different approach, some doctors treated the thymus region of psoriasis patients with X-rays rather than the skin lesions themselves (cited in Ref 6). It is not clear what the rationale was for this; perhaps this was an attempt to correct the internal defect that they believed to underlie psoriasis. Galowski treated 82 cases, 14 of which were cleared whilst 40 showed improvement. Only 2 of the cases got worse, 5 were unaffected and the remaining 21 were not followed up. In contrast, Brock observed only 2 patients whose skin resolved and a few that showed improvement in the large number of cases that he treated using the same rationale.

In common with treatments used today, the benefits of X-rays in the treatment of psoriasis did not come without a price. If the dose given was too large, or if large areas were exposed at a given time, as in cases of extensive psoriasis, serious toxic side effects could result. Thus it was essential that both the patient and doctor were protected from inappropriate exposure. At a meeting of the New York Dermatological Society to discuss the use of X-rays in psoriasis in December 1920[7], it was concluded that the therapy was safe and efficacious if practised by dermatologists who had both knowledge of the disease and experience in the use of roentgen therapy. Subsequently, advances in the degree of protection against radiation and in the accuracy of measurement of doses considerably reduced the hazards of X-ray therapy, which continued to be used for the treatment of psoriasis until the 1980s.

Soon after Roentgen received his Nobel Prize for the discovery of X-rays in 1901, Marie and Pierre Curie successfully purified a sample of radium, a radioactive product of uranium. Radium was immediately used to treat cancer, but, in common with X-rays, its harmful effects (including burning of the skin, respiratory problems and damage to the bone marrow leading to cancers) tempered its therapeutic applications. Radcliffe Crocker was the first dermatologist to use radium to treat skin diseases, including plaque psoriasis[8]. He used the emanations given off from a solution of radium bromide, which were held in solution in water and administered topically in a weak gelatin jelly, (or by subcutaneous injection in cases of mycosis fungoides). The freshly prepared jelly was melted and applied to lesional skin, then covered with muslin, followed by lead foil that was bandaged on to prevent loss of the gamma rays. A better therapeutic effect was observed the longer the jelly was left on the skin and no adverse side effects were observed after 12 hours, resulting in clearance of hard patches of a psoriasis on the knees of a 12 year old girl which remained clear for a year or more. However, radium was expensive and difficult to obtain which limited its use as a therapeutic agent in psoriasis.

A third type of radiation, the so-called "infra-roentgen" or "grenz rays", was also used, although to a lesser extent, for the treatment of psoriasis[9]. Grenz rays, from the German word grenze meaning border, are a low energy radiation present in the zone between X-rays and short wavelength ultraviolet (UV) radiation, which were discovered in 1925 by Gustav Bucky. Grenz rays have a low penetration of about 2mm, which restricts their use to the treatment of skin diseases. In those cases that respond to its effects, the results are rapid (48-72 hours) and the procedure relatively safe and painless as there is no damage to underlying structures of the skin. Grenz ray treatment was used for many years in Europe and Scandinavia, but was not favoured in America, although its use increased later when improvements to the design of the tubes were made, and more accurate measurement of doses became possible.

Phototherapy

The first therapeutic use of sunlight (heliotherapy) in skin diseases was probably in 1400 BC. By the beginning of the 20th century, heliotherapy with natural sunlight was mainly used in thermal stations to treat tuberculosis and, during World War I, to treat leg ulcers. The existence of UV wavelengths or nonvisible "chemical rays" had been demonstrated in 1801, but it wasn't until the end of the 19th century that it was realised that it was these rays that exerted the majority of the therapeutic effects of sunlight. This led to the first use of artificial light sources for the treatment of skin diseases (phototherapy).

In 1903, Finsen in Copenhagen was awarded the Nobel Prize in Medicine, the only dermatologist to have received one, for the successful treatment of lupus (vulgaris) with concentrated doses of UV radiation from a carbon arc lamp. By 1905, phototherapy was beginning to be used to treat various other skin conditions, including eczema, acne and psoriasis. Subsequently, smaller and relatively inexpensive mercury vapor quartz UV lamps also became available. In Europe, dermatologists used either carbon arc or quartz mercury lamps, but in America, Finsen's carbon arc lamp was not used for economical reasons. The carbon arc lamps provided intense UV light with a spectrum approximately that of the sun, and, in addition, emitted infrared rays in large quantities, which added to the efficacy of the treatment. In contrast, the quartz mercury arc generators produced shorter,

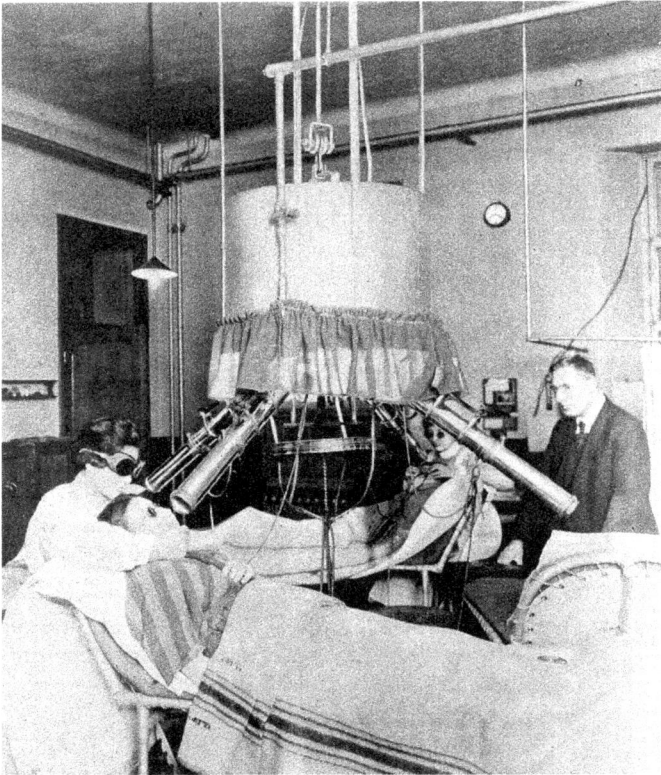

Guy's Hospital Bicentenary: Finsen lamp treatment. From the Illustrated London News, Jan-Jun 1925. Wellcome Library, London.

29

more effective wavelengths. In addition, as less heat was produced, the source could be put closer to the skin resulting in shorter exposure times. Both types of lamps gave equally beneficial effects and were successfully used to treat a large number of psoriasis patients.

Psoriasis was treated in either of two ways; frequent general whole body irradiation, or irradiation of circumscribed eruptions or lesions. Whole body irradiation, produced by large air-cooled UV lamps, involved doses too small to evoke erythema (redness), and aimed to influence the disease via possible systemic effects. Irradiation of distinct lesions, on the other hand, used erythema and blistering-inducing doses; these were not repeated until all evidence of a reaction had disappeared. This latter approach was not particularly effective and only sometimes induced resolution when applied once a week. Daily whole body irradiation was, however, considered by many dermatologists to be of benefit. Remission times were longer than that obtained with X-rays, and, in addition, UV light was more suitable for treatment of the scalp than X-rays, which often caused the hair to drop out.

Importantly, in 1919 it was demonstrated that UV from mercury quartz lamps (or cod liver oil) could prevent or treat rickets, a disease that was not uncommon amongst urban children at the beginning of the 20th century. This was later shown to be due to the synthesis of vitamin D in the skin when subjected to UV irradiation. This led to the use of vitamin D, and much later, vitamin D analogues, in the treatment of psoriasis.

The Goeckerman treatment

In 1925, a new treatment for severe psoriasis was introduced by Goeckerman, which combined UV irradiation with crude coal tar[10]. The development of this treatment was arrived at by chance, resulting from Goeckerman's idea of sensitising skin plaques artificially to UV light in order to speed up resolution. He tried various fluorescent compounds, some of which were known to be photosensitising, but without effect. In contrast when he tried crude coal tar, chosen because of its complexity, it was almost immediately successful. However, Goeckerman realised that its therapeutic efficacy was probably not due to a photosensitising effect.

The Goeckerman treatment involved the application of tar ointment three times a day, followed the next day by the removal of excess tar with vegetable oil prior to UV irradiation with a hot quartz lamp. The oil, tar and scales were then washed off in a soap tub bath before reapplication of fresh tar ointment. The nature of this procedure meant that it was necessary for patients to be hospitalised, although a modification of the method allowed its use on an outpatient basis. The treatment lasted on average for 2-3 weeks for moderate cases, and 3-4 weeks for severe cases. Of 181 patients treated by Goeckerman between 1925 and 1930, only 3 patients failed to respond to the treatment. Furthermore, the treatment was equally successful for generalised exfoliative psoriasis as for chronic plaque psoriasis. The number of patients treated at the Mayo Clinic, Rochester, Minnesota[11] subsequently increased steadily to 250-300 per year in the 1980s. However, many dermatologists (and patients) did not embrace this approach to treatment with the same enthusiasm, finding the procedure too messy and time-consuming.

Anthralin

As mentioned in Chapter 2, chrysarobin derived from the araroba tree was used to treat psoriasis during the 19th century and its use continued into the early 1900s. However, during World War I it became difficult to import it to Germany from Brazil, and supplies became depleted. Thus, Galewsky, a dermatologist living and working in Dresden, Saxony, requested the Bayer Company to synthesise a substance similar in structure to chrysarobin (anthralin), which he named "Cignolin". In 1916, he published his clinical findings which showed that the most effective anti-psoriatic formulation contained 0.05% to 0.1% anthralin in acetone, or included 0.5% salicyclic acid and liquor carbonis detergens in an ointment base[12]. At the same time, Unna tested several derivatives of

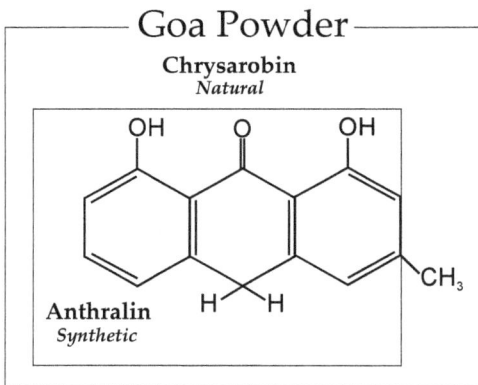

Goa Powder

Chrysarobin
Natural

Anthralin
Synthetic

anthrone, and found that only anthralin and 1-hydroxy, 9-anthrone had anti-psoriatic properties[13]. Initially, anthralin was not widely accepted, leading the manufacturer to stop production both in 1924 and 1929. However, subsequent reports were favourable and most authors found that the synthetic anthralin was more effective than the natural product, chrysarobin. Unfortunately, the efficacy of anthralin and its side effects of irritation and staining were closely related. Since that time, anthralin (also known as dithranol) has remained the most effective anthrone derivative for the treatment of psoriasis.

Myelocene: a bone marrow preparation

In 1902, a preparation of bone marrow named "myelocene" diluted in almond oil was used to directly treat the psoriatic skin lesions of 5 patients[14]. This substance, which had been prepared by extracting the marrow from animal bones with ether and then evaporating to produce a fatty product, had previously been used to treat a series of patients with chronic ear disease. The reason for its use in psoriasis is not, therefore, immediately apparent! However, the ability of bone marrow to produce "a substance that is a powerful prophylactic against various bacteria found in various sites throughout the body" was cited, suggesting that this may have been the basis for its use in psoriasis. Treatment with myelocene was claimed to reduce irritation and induce resolution of skin lesions even at sites to which the substance had not been applied. However, there was variability in effectiveness between different preparations, and care was required in administration of the substance. It seems incredible now that such a prestigious medical journal as the Lancet should have published these findings, but it is an example of the "try-it-and-see" approach to the treatment of psoriasis which dominated at this time.

The advances in scientific knowledge at the beginning of the 20th century led to novel approaches to the treatment of psoriasis. No further progress in the development of effective therapies was to emerge until the middle of the century when the use of topical glucocorticoids was to mark a new era in the treatment of skin diseases (Chapter 6).

~ 4 ~

The 1930s

During the 1930s, the microbial hypothesis for psoriasis continued to be favoured by some dermatologists, with further observations of a bacillus in skin lesions, and some evidence of a link with a preceding tonsillitis. The association of psoriasis with arthritis became more established, and attempts were made to define psoriatic arthritis as a separate entity. No major new treatments were developed during this period, although various approaches, such as the administration of vitamin D, adrenal cortex extracts and ACTH and, in Russia, the use of lysates prepared from body organs, were tried with variable success.

Bacteria, psoriasis and arthritis

An association between psoriasis and arthritis had been recognised since the 19th century. Considerable variation in the clinical presentation of psoriasis-associated arthritis was observed, and so attempts were made to define the so-called "psoriasis arthropica" as a definite entity in order to exclude any coincidental association. The definition included the simultaneous waxing and waning of the two conditions, the arthritic involvement of the terminal interphalangeal joints (between the end and middle finger bones), and pitting of the nails of the fingers and toes.

During the 1930s, the relationship between psoriasis and arthritis was examined in more detail, in particular with regard to the role of microorganisms in both diseases. At this time, research work in different parts of the world had indicated that the causal organism in rheumatic infection was a streptococcus. A relationship between the presence of *Streptococcus haemolyticus* in the upper respiratory tract and rheumatic symptoms was suggested by the disappearance of both when patients transferred from New York to Porto Rico, a place where the organism was not prevalent, and reappeared again with a return to New York. Furthermore, lesions similar to subcutaneous nodules present in the skin and heart of patients with acute rheumatic fever could be produced experimentally in animals by injection of streptococci. It was concluded from these animal studies that allergy, a term introduced in 1906 by von Pirquet to describe

33

the change in reactivity that occurs after the first exposure to an antigen, played an important role in the formation of rheumatic nodules.

In a report in the Lancet in 1933, Elizabeth Hunt discussed the similarities between psoriasis and rheumatic infections[1]. She observed that half of her series of 53 cases of psoriasis gave a history of tonsillitis or sore throats. Furthermore, 70% of these were experiencing rheumatic symptoms, and 80% gave a familial history of some form of rheumatic infection. In addition, the similarity between the histological features present in psoriatic skin lesions and the subcutaneous nodules of acute rheumatism also supported a link between the two conditions. Based upon these findings, together with the observation that psoriasis and allergic conditions share similar clinical features, she proposed that psoriasis was a non-specific allergic reaction of the skin.

The idea that psoriasis may be mediated by non-specific allergic reactions to various antigens, and that consideration of the possible provoking factors in each patient should be taken into account before treatment, was emphasised by Barber in a letter to the Editor a few years later in the same journal[2]. He supported this hypothesis with the following clinical observations. In the majority of cases of psoriasis appearing for the first time in childhood, he noted an association with a preceding haemolytic streptococci infection (tonsillitis or scarlet fever). Effective treatment of the infection led to resolution of the psoriasis, suggesting a causative link. However, in patients in whom psoriasis started for the first time in adult life, a variety of provoking factors were implicated (including streptococcal and other bacterial infections), as also observed in adults with rheumatism.

One such aetiological factor identified at this time was *Bacillus endoparasiticus,* a spore-forming bacillus detected by Tibor Benedek in the blood and skin of psoriatic patients[3]. The bacillus was often observed in the connective tissue surrounding the sweat or sebaceous glands in the dermis of psoriatic skin lesions. A previous study in 1910 had identified a "short, stumpy" bacillus in psoriatic skin lesions (see Chapter 3), but whether this was the same organism is not known. Benedek's findings were not confirmed by other researchers, which was suggested by the author to be due to the choice of stain employed in other studies. Benedek used Weigert's lithium carmine stain, and noted that, when inflammation was severe, the number of organisms was small, whilst numerous endoparasites were observed in the connective tissue of skin lesions showing only moderate inflammation.

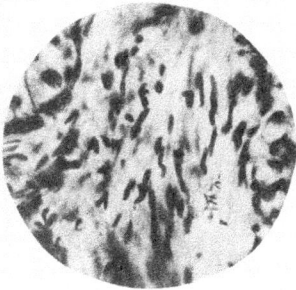

Fig. 4. B. endoparasiticus, S type, in the stratum re-
ticulare of a psoriatic lesion. Numerous parasites are
in the periglandular connective tissue of a sebaceous
gland.

*Benedek T, 1955. Wellcome
Library, London*

Benedek interpreted these findings as showing that the "psoriatic lesion is the result of an interplay between host and endoparasite in the presence of a specific constitution of the individual".

Normal as well as psoriatic individuals mounted a tuberculosis-type delayed hypersensitivity reaction to skin testing with a vaccine of the bacillus, suggesting that they had also been exposed to the organism. Furthermore, the bacillus was associated with other skin diseases such as seborrheic dermatitis, pityriasis rosea and pompholyx. It was suggested that these differences in clinical presentation might result from differences in the intensity of the bacteraemia, location of the eruption, or "disposition" of the skin. The additional presence of the bacillus in the joints of patients with rheumatoid (psoriatic) arthritis prompted Benedek to suggest that an allergic inflammatory process to the bacillus in connective tissue formed the basis of a common aetiology shared by psoriasis and its associated arthritis. Attempts to resolve psoriasis by vaccination with the bacillus were, however, unsuccessful. Indeed, higher concentrations of the vaccine induced exacerbation of the disease.

The bacillus observed by Benedek was, some 40 years later, identified as *Bacillus licheniformis*, an organism commonly present in the blood of normal individuals. It seems likely that its presence in the skin and joints of psoriasis patients can be explained by migration from the blood during the inflammatory process, and is, therefore, probably secondary to the disease rather than causative.

In addition to studies of the role of environmental factors in the aetiology of psoriasis, the hereditary nature of the disease was also being investigated. A comparison of the incidence of psoriasis in monozygotic or identical (10 of 15) and dizygotic or non-identical (2 of 12) twins, provided the first evidence to support the long held belief that psoriasis had a strong genetic component. Studies of the immediate families of psoriasis patients did not, however, support either a recessive or dominant inheritance i.e.

35

two faulty recessive genes or a single dominant faulty gene required for expression, respectively. This suggests that there were differences in the penetrance of the psoriasis gene(s), so that it was not always expressed. In 1931, Hoede published the findings of an extensive analysis of psoriasis patients, which included a genetic analysis of psoriatic pedigrees collected by him during the previous 5 years[4]. However he came to different conclusions concerning the nature of genetic inheritance, namely that "psoriasis is an irregular dominant, which is incompletely sex-limited", a theory which is not supported by current findings.

Treatments

Treatments introduced at the beginning of the 20th century, such as X-rays, UV light and anthralin, and the more established treatments such as arsenic, mercury and tars, continued to be used as the century progressed. In England, Ingram introduced a new approach to the use of anthralin for the treatment of psoriasis by combining it with UV light. Various other treatments were tried with varying success, including the administration of vitamins (B1, C and D), adrenal cortex extracts or ACTH, and undecylinic acid.

Ingram's regimen

This treatment approach was similar to that of Goeckerman, except that anthralin was substituted for crude coal tar. Ingram's regimen involved the patient soaking in a bath with added coal tar solution, then exposure to increasing UV light doses to maintain near erythema dose, and finally application of anthralin in Lassar's paste to lesional skin alone. This was left on for 24 hours under stockinet and then removed prior to bathing with olive oil. The preparation of anthralin in Lassar's paste (consisting of petrolatum, salicylic acid, zinc oxide and starch) was an essential development as it prevented the drug from spreading and irritating non-lesional skin. The stiffness of the paste was determined by the melting point of the petrolatum and could be further increased by the addition of paraffin wax. The presence of the salicylic acid was required to prevent alkaline oxidation of anthralin from impurities in the zinc oxide, and also acted as a mild keratolytic. The treatment underwent various modifications and proved to be as successful as that of Goeckerman's regimen.

Vitamin D

The relationship between UV light exposure, increased vitamin D production and resolution of psoriatic skin lesions was observed in 1936. This resulted in the administration of vitamin D both orally and topically, either as a synthetic preparation or in fish oils. Topical application of vitamin D proved to be ineffective, whilst some success was observed with oral preparations. Thus one study showed that daily treatment with large doses of vitamin D induced complete resolution of skin lesions in 11 of 15 patients with chronic, widespread psoriasis within 12 weeks of treatment[5]. The disease subsequently relapsed in 6 patients after 6 weeks to 5 months, whilst 4 patients remained disease-free for 3-8 months. However, such success with vitamin D treatment was not reproduced by other dermatologists. In addition, the therapy was associated with hypercalcaemic side effects such as nausea, diarrhoea, polyurea and weight loss, which resulted in vitamin D treatment for psoriasis being discontinued in the 1940s. Interestingly, the moderate beneficial effects of the vitamin in psoriasis (at least in some patients) was to be "rediscovered" approximately 50 years later in a patient treated with a vitamin D analogue for osteoporosis. This led to the revival of the use of vitamin D as a therapeutic tool for psoriasis.

Adrenal cortex extracts/ACTH

In Germany, Gruneberg proposed that psoriasis was caused by hypofunction of the adrenal cortex in psoriasis and proceeded to publish several papers during this period on the effects of treating psoriasis patients with adrenal cortex extracts (Cortidyn) or adrenocorticotropic hormone (ACTH), a hormone produced by the pituitary gland that stimulates secretion of adrenal cortical steroids. Cortidyn was a clear, yellowish liquid containing gamma adrenalin, 1 cc of which was equivalent to 50 grams of fresh cortical tissue. Patients were injected intravenously or intramuscularly with 2-3 cc of the extract daily for several weeks, the only side effects being occasional headaches. Approximately one-fifth of the patients were cleared, whilst three-fifths improved to varying extents. Although beneficial effects were seen within a few days (more rapidly the higher the dose), this could cease suddenly without further improvement, thus local treatment was also required. In addition, relapse often occurred promptly when treatment was stopped. The best results were seen in patients with severe psoriasis and arthritis who had failed to improve with other therapies. However, after treating 200 psoriasis patients with Cortidyn, Gruneberg still wasn't able to prove or disprove his theory of the dysfunction of the adrenal glands as a cause of psoriasis.

Gruneberg also treated 30 psoriasis patients with 1-4 cc per day of ACTH, which was equivalent to 0.3-1.2 grams of fresh glandular tissue. Again resolution started in the first week of treatment, but was preceded by exacerbation within the first couple of days, a phenomenon that has also been observed with current treatments such as PUVA (psoralens plus UV light). Generally, better therapeutic effects were seen in psoriasis with ACTH than with adrenal cortex extracts.

Following on from these and earlier attempts to treat psoriasis systemically with metabolic extracts and hormones, the treatment of skin diseases was revolutionised at the beginning of the 1950s with the development of topical glucocorticosteroids (see Chapter 5).

Undecylinic acid

As is the case today, reports of new treatments by the media stimulated numerous enquiries by psoriasis patients searching for a more effective remedy. For example, the success of a small uncontrolled study of psoriasis patients with the anti-fungal drug, undecylinic acid, prompted requests by patients attending St John's Hospital for Diseases of the Skin in London for "the new American treatment". This resulted in comprehensive trials being carried out with the drug to test its efficacy[6]. Some cases were treated as inpatients at the Middlesex Hospital, whilst others attended an outpatient clinic at St John's Hospital. They were given either undecylinic acid capsules, capsules containing a placebo (inert oil), or calciferol (vitamin D). Those patients who were using local applications at the time continued to do so, whilst those that weren't received the oral medication only. The findings showed a moderate effect by calciferol, but little evidence of any beneficial effect exerted by undecylinic acid over a 8 week period. This was in agreement with several other reports of the use of undecylinic acid in psoriasis, and illustrated the importance of carrying out controlled studies of large numbers of patients to determine treatment efficacy.

Tissue lysates

In Russia, the "wonder" treatment of this period consisted of lysates prepared by proteolytic enzyme hydrolysis of body organs in an acid medium under high pressure, which were used to treat various diseases in humans and animals. The lysates were claimed to have specific effects on the organs from which they were prepared, although many Russian scientists at the time doubted the validity of this claim. One of the people treated with these lysates by Dr Idnaty Kazakow was reputed to be Joseph Stalin, who, in addition to his other ailments, appeared to suffer from psoriasis[7]. An initial treatment cleared his skin, but later an exacerbation of disease activity resulting in pigmentary skin changes was unresponsive to a second treatment of the lysates. The initial success of Kazakow's lysate treatment in a small group of important people resulted in his being given substantial professional support, and large sums of money to hire additional staff and buy modern equipment to continue his research. However, the failure of Stalin's lysate treatment had serious consequences for Kazakow who, along with other doctors, was charged of crimes covered by the Anti-Soviet Article 58 of the criminal code (including murder) in the "great trials" in Moscow in 1938. He defended his lysate therapy and maintained it was harmless; however, it was not enough to save him from execution.

~ 5~

Pre-war Germany and World War II

Nazi removal of Jewish doctors and dermatologists

In Germany the removal of Jewish doctors from medical boards and committees, and from editorial boards of the most prestigious medical journals, started in 1933 and included probably the most famous dermatologist in the world at this time, Joseph Jadassohn (reviewed in Ref 1). Dermatology had been established in Germany as a medical speciality primarily by Jews, and the Nazi regime attempted to conceal this fact by replacing those in prominent positions with Nazi representatives and banning any reference to their work in publications. Anything that celebrated the achievements of Jewish doctors, such as the bust of Paul Unna at the skin clinic of Hamburg University, was hidden or destroyed. Collaboration with other dermatologists in countries such as the Netherlands and Czechoslovakia ceased and the quality of clinical and research publications declined. Eventually Jewish physicians were removed from the practice of medicine completely, being arrested in hospitals and taken away to be tortured and beaten to death. It was estimated that as many as 5% of Jewish doctors living in Germany, amounting to several hundred, committed suicide at this time. By 1936, 458 Jewish physicians (23 of which were dermatologists) were ousted from German Universities, with the largest number of professorial chairs coming from departments of Dermatology. Many Jewish dermatologists fled to America where they played a substantial role in the development of the speciality; few ever returned to their native countries.

Eugenics and psoriasis

When the Nazis took power, they introduced The Law for the Prevention of Genetically Diseased Offspring in July 1933, which provided a legal basis for the compulsory sterilisation of the mentally ill and disabled. This was in line with the Nazi policy of enhancing the genetic quality of the human race by restricting the birth rate of the "unfit" and encouraging reproduction of the "fit" (eugenics). Surprisingly, a similar law had been

41

passed in 1907 in Indiana, USA allowing compulsory sterilisation of the mentally ill and criminally insane, and by the late 1920s, 28 states in America and one province in Canada had enacted the legislation resulting in the sterilisation of some 15,000 men and women.

At this time a dermatologist at the University of Würzburg, Karl Hoede, was pursuing his interest in the genetic aspects of cutaneous diseases, especially psoriasis. Hoede thought that skin diseases should be included under this law of eugenics, and he therefore proposed that they should be classified according to the extent of their inheritability. Thus any skin disease predominantly caused by genetic factors, such as xeroderma pigmentosum or epidermal bullosa, and congenital hyperkeratoses should be subject to the law. However, for other conditions with "substantial" genetic influence, including certain types of eczema and psoriasis, he did not go as far as to advocate enforced sterilisation but stated that "a decision is badly needed to clarify in which patients with cutaneous diseases marriage is not in the best interests of the people". Other dermatologists, such as Leo van Zumbusch, who had described in 1910 what is now known as generalised pustular psoriasis (van Zumbusch disease), were ardent anti-Nazis. He was confined to his home during the Nazi period in Germany in what was the equivalent to house–arrest, and died in 1940, thus avoiding the inevitable fate of incarceration and subsequent death in a concentration camp.

Psoriasis and the military in World War II

Although usually not life-threatening, skin diseases in general have proved to be a significant problem in military operations because they are a significant cause of combat ineffectiveness, morbidity and poor morale. During WWII, a lack of specialised dermatology training by medical officers resulted in inaccurate diagnosis and inappropriate treatment of skin disorders thus exacerbating the problem. Indeed, over half of the man-days lost to frontline troops were directly related to common skin diseases such as psoriasis. This situation hadn't changed since WWI when psoriasis followed impetigo, scabies, boils and pediculosis as the most frequent reasons for dermatology admissions in a British general hospital between November 1915 and June 1916[2]. The natural history of psoriasis with its fluctuating activity, tendency to be exacerbated by certain stimuli, and chronicity led to approximately 20% of psoriasis patients becoming unfit to participate in military combat during WWII. Flare-up of skin lesions were caused by various factors including transfer to a cold climate or hostile environment, anti-malarial chemoprophylaxis (administration of chloroquin), and the stress and anxiety that accompanied training and subsequent deployment to war zones. In addition, the onset of psoriasis was observed as a sequel to wounding, with lesions developing near wounds or in the subsequent scar.

At the end of the war, military personnel provided an accessible source of patients for the study of the aetiology of psoriasis. In one study, the role of psychological factors in 86 military patients with psoriasis were investigated, the previous personality of 72 of which was assessed by psychiatric examination[3]. Twenty-nine were classed as emotionally well adjusted, and 43 as maladjusted, the latter showing either definite personality deviations before the onset of skin lesions or psychiatric symptoms at the time of onset. This number of maladjusted individuals far exceeded a random sample of soldiers. Emotional factors were implicated in the aetiology of the disease in 49 of the psoriatics, which, in approximately half of the cases, were unrelated to any psychological problems they may have been experiencing. Clearly the social effects of having a disease such as psoriasis whilst serving in the military were especially distressing. Communal life necessitated undressing in front of other soldiers prompting unkind comments and (ungrounded) fears of catching the disease. This caused anxiety about their condition and the need to cover up their affected skin as much as possible, leading to a fear of bath parades, withdrawal from sporting activities and also, in some cases, from social occasions. These worries extended to their personal lives, affecting their relationships with women and concern about whether the disease will be passed onto their children.

All of these considerations, including the side effects often experienced during treatment with systemic medicines, have led to a bar on patients with psoriasis, or a history of psoriasis joining the British Army today, although the conditions are less stringent for joining the Royal Navy or Royal Air Force.

Nutrition and psoriasis

It has been a common belief that psoriasis improves under conditions of poor nutrition, as experienced during a time of war. A report by Simons published in 1949, which described the effects on psoriasis of the internment of Dutch individuals in Japanese concentration camps in Java

43

during WWII, has been frequently cited in support of this[4]. However, reconsideration of the results of Simons' study by Zackheim and Farber calls this premise into question[5]. Thus of the 13 individuals studied, only seven improved (two only slightly) and two others showed only transient improvement. Two patients became worse, whilst two others showed no change in their disease. Interestingly, the relapse observed in two patients after initial improvement coincided with heavy fatigue duty or depression. However, as noted by Simons, the patients were forced to work practically naked in direct sunlight. Such exposure to UV light would be sufficient to explain the resolution of disease seen in some of the patients, making it difficult to assess the contribution of poor nutrition.

Other authors have failed to find a relationship between improvement of psoriasis and poor nutrition. For example, Gans found no association between the incidence of psoriasis in Germany, and the periods encompassing the two World Wars when nutrition was poor[6]. In contrast, Simons noted in his report that a study by Prakken found that psoriasis got worse in 53 of 99 cases in the Netherlands in 1942, despite (or because of?) low fat rations.

In an attempt to determine the true relationship between psoriasis and changes in diet, Zackheim and Farber carried out a study in which the effect of a weight-reducing 500 calorie diet was compared to that of a regular diet in hospitalized patients for three to five weeks[5]. Half of the patients on a regular diet (4/8) improved, whilst two were unchanged and two became worse. In contrast, seven of the eight patients on the low calorie diet became worse, whilst the remaining patient improved slightly. A regular diet followed by a low calorie diet in two patients confirmed that the latter was associated with exacerbation of the disease. Thus, the evidence available at this time was not consistent with a beneficial effect of poor nutrition on psoriasis. Indeed quite the opposite; it pointed towards a detrimental effect on disease progression.

Interestingly, it had been previously proposed by Grütz and Bürger in 1933 that psoriasis was caused by a disturbance in the metabolism of fats[7]. This was based upon clinical studies in which fasting individuals were given cholesterin (cholesterol) in olive oil, then blood was taken three times over the next 24 hours so that serum fat and lipid levels could be determined. The total fat content was found to be, on average, 40% higher in psoriatics than normal individuals, and there was also an increase in cholesterin and phosphatide compounds. On the basis of these results, it was recommended that dairy products such as cream, butter and cheese should be banned from the psoriatics' diet, and that fat intake in an adult patient should be reduced to a maximum of 20g/ day. However, although this approach did prove beneficial in some cases (in common with many other treatments for psoriasis) the hypothesis was not proven and the low-fat diet was later abandoned.

Development of anti-bacterial treatments

Intensive efforts were being made in the early 1930s to find compounds with anti-bacterial activity. The demonstration that certain sulfonamides exhibited anti-bacterial potential was made by Gerhard Domagk in Germany, and led to the introduction of "Prontosil" on to the market in 1935. As a result of this work, Domagk was subsequently awarded the Nobel Prize for Medicine and Physiology, but was not permitted to accept it by the National Socialists of pre-war Germany. He was not to receive the diploma and medal until 1949. Further compounds of similar structure were subsequently investigated for possible anti-bacterial activity, including diaminodiphenylsulfone (dapsone), which had been first synthesised at the turn of the century. Dapsone was tested out on Jewish internees by Vonkennel (University of Leipzig) at the concentration camp in Buchenwald in gruesome experiments in which they were subjected to poison gas, inducing severe burns, many of them dying in the process. Vonkennel, who was also the director of the SS Research Institute V, ran the only skin clinic in Germany whose research was still being funded by the Nazi government.

In the early 1940s, dapsone and related sulfones gained worldwide recognition for treating leprosy and other infectious diseases. On this basis, dapsone was given to patients with dermatitis herpetiformis (DH) in 1950, on the erroneous assumption that it was an infectious skin disease. Surprisingly the drug proved to be very effective, and is currently used not only for DH, but for other non-infectious inflammatory, autoimmune and bullous skin diseases, including pustular psoriasis.

Although dapsone is still used to treat leprosy, a major development in medicine at this time was to supersede its use in other infections caused by microorganisms such as streptococci, pneumococci, diphtheria bacilli and syphilis. This was the availability of penicillin, whose use during the war saved the lives of thousands of wounded soldiers who would have succumbed to subsequent infections. Penicillin was discovered by chance in 1928 by Alexander Fleming, a microbiologist at St Mary's Hospital, London,

45

who noticed the disappearance of colonies of staphylococci adjacent to a mould that had contaminated the plate. However, it wasn't until Ernst Boris Chain, a refugee from Nazi Germany and his boss, Howard Walter Florey in Oxford carried out research on the anti-microbial effects of the fungus-derived product, and initiated its commercial production, that large amounts of the antibiotic became available. In recognition of their work, Fleming, Florey and Chain shared the Nobel Prize for Medicine at the end of the war.

The discovery of penicillin had implications for patients with various diseases caused or exacerbated by bacteria, including skin diseases such as psoriasis. Circumstantial evidence for the triggering of acute psoriasis by a streptococcal throat infection had been reported in the previous decade. A further observation was made in 1945 that supported a causal relationship between streptococci and psoriasis[8]. This was the marked sensitivity shown by psoriasis patients to skin injections of minute amounts of a vaccine of a certain strain of *Streptococcus faecalis*, isolated from the patients, which resulted in the formation of a psoriatic lesion at the site of injection and worsening of pre-existing psoriasis. In contrast, injection of the streptococcal vaccine in smaller doses sometimes resulted in improvement. The first definitive evidence of the presence of a streptococcal infection in psoriasis patients prior to a skin eruption was to be published in the decade following the war (see Chapter 6).

~ 6 ~

The 1950s

During the period after the Second World War, some clues as to the nature of the aetiology of the psoriasis began to emerge. Statistical genetic analyses of psoriasis patients and their families led to a new hypothesis proposing that at least 2 genes were involved in the predisposition to develop psoriasis, and, evidence that confirmed a relationship between acute guttate psoriasis and a prior streptococcal throat infection was reported. In addition, the development of the Rose-Waaler test made it possible to differentiate rheumatoid arthritis from psoriatic arthritis, so that the various manifestations of the latter could be more clearly defined.

This period was also of importance because it marked the start of a new era in the treatment of psoriasis, the use of drugs based on their mechanism of action; anti-inflammatory topical glucocorticosteroids and the anti-metabolites, aminopterin and methotrexate.

Aetiology: Genetics

The general consensus at this time was that a predisposition to psoriasis was inherited via a dominant gene with reduced penetrance (reviewed in reference 1). That is, in some individuals who carry the disease gene, the disease is not expressed. Further Hoede claimed that this dominant gene was incompletely sex-limited (see Chapter 4). However, a statistical genetic analysis of 464 unselected patients and their parents, children and siblings published in 1951 came to different conclusions[2]. No relationship was found between the sex of the patient, parents and siblings ruling out the possibility of sex-linked inheritance. Furthermore, it was found that psoriasis occurred amongst the patients' siblings with a frequency of 9% when one parent was affected, compared to only a 2.45% frequency when neither parent had psoriasis. It was argued that a single gene hypothesis, whether it was dominant (one copy required for disease expression) or recessive (2 copies required for disease expression), with or without complete penetrance, was not consistent with these findings. It was therefore proposed that a minimum of 2 genes was likely to be involved in the predisposition of an individual to psoriasis. One possibility put

47

forward, for which there was some preliminary statistical evidence, was that psoriatic patients carried 2 unlinked recessive genes on non-sex chromosomes. In each case, 2 copies of each gene were present, allowing disease expression. This was the first report suggesting that there was likely to be more than one gene involved in psoriasis susceptibility, a hypothesis that, more than 50 years on, is supported by extensive evidence.

Aetiology: Streptococci

During the 1930s, there had been preliminary reports of cases in which psoriasis eruptions occurred in association with infections of the throat. In the following decade, it became possible to obtain evidence for a streptococcal infection, past or present, by measurement of the level of serum antibodies to streptolysin O (ASO titres), a toxin released by the bacteria which causes complete lysis of red blood cells in blood agar plates. Norrlind was the first to use this test to investigate whether patients with widespread, sudden eruptions of mainly guttate psoriasis showed evidence of a prior infection by β haemolytic streptococci[3]. Of 32 such patients attending the Clinic of Dermatology and Venereology in Lund, Sweden, 18 (56%) had raised ASO titres. Of these 18, 10 gave histories

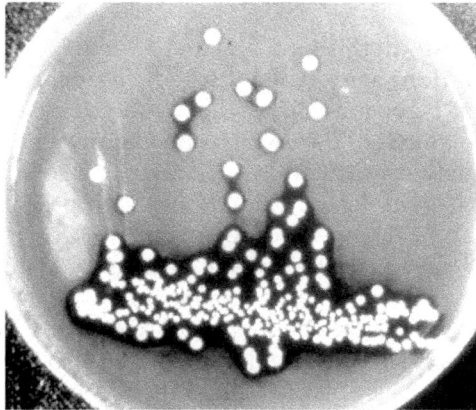

Red cell lysis around colonies of streptococci on a blood agar plate. Courtesy of Professor S. Joseph, University of Maryland, and Dr David Rollins, Naval Medical Research Center, Bethesda, USA.

of infections of the throat and upper respiratory tract 1-3 weeks before the appearance of skin lesions. Furthermore, in 7 of the 18, β haemolytic streptococci were grown from throat swabs.

Similar results were obtained by Norrlind in a further set of 65 cases[3] and were confirmed by Norholm-Pedersen in Denmark in a study of 133 guttate and/or plaque psoriasis patients, one-third of which showed raised ASO titres[4]. Raised antibody titres were more frequent in younger patients and in women rather than men, and were associated with guttate psoriasis, often with the first eruption of skin lesions. The degree of elevation of the ASO titre did not appear to be associated with the extent of skin lesions or their response to treatment. However, administration of penicillin was found to be helpful in some cases, to prevent further skin flares or to increase response to topical treatments, when the provoking streptococcal infection was persistent or recurrent.

Although the original case report (in 1916) that related acute psoriasis to a preceding tonsillitis was made by an American, this was not followed up in American psoriasis patients until 10 years after the observations made by the Scandinavian authors[5]. The findings confirmed those previously reported in patients with acute guttate psoriasis, and two possible mechanisms for the initiation of psoriasis as a sequel to a streptococcal infection were proposed. The first proposal was that toxins produced by the bacteria induced capillary changes in the dermal layer of the skin. Dermal capillaries are known to be susceptible to the effects of streptococcal erythrogenic toxin, and in trauma-induced psoriasis (the Koebner reaction), capillary alterations precede epidermal changes, which would be consistent with the delay between the onset of the infection and the appearance of skin lesions. The second hypothesis suggested that psoriasis resulted from an allergic antibody response to either streptococcal products or host tissue combined with, or altered by, a streptococcal product. A hypersensitivity response to streptococci, which was presumed to be involved in post-streptococcal sequelae such as acute rheumatic fever and acute glomerulonephritis, was considered to be a less likely explanation due to the absence of systemic symptoms in psoriasis patients.

This report also contained the findings of one of the first uses of tonsillectomy to treat psoriasis patients with persistent or recurrent streptococcal infections. Removal of the tonsils resulted in markedly reduced ASO titres and, although occasional plaques of psoriasis sometimes appeared subsequently, the patients responded well to treatment.

Arthritis

Since the 19th century, various rheumatic complaints had been reported to be associated with psoriasis, particularly that of rheumatoid arthritis (RA). Some dermatologists regarded this as merely a chance coincidence, whilst others believed that true "psoriatic arthropathy" could be defined by a strict set of criteria. However, many of the rheumatic symptoms experienced by psoriatic patients failed to meet these criteria. With the introduction of the Rose-Waaler (RW) sheep cell agglutination test, it became possible to differentiate RA (RW-positive in approximately 80% of patients) from the other types of arthritis observed in psoriasis patients (RW-negative). The RW test measured the presence of "rheumatoid factor", an antibody produced in patients with RA that is directed against the IgG (immunoglobulin G) type of antibody, which causes agglutination of sheep red blood cells coated in IgG antiserum.

Using this test, together with clinical observations, Wright carried out a re-evaluation of 154 psoriatic patients with rheumatic symptoms[6]. Twenty-three of the patients were diagnosed with osteoarthritis, gout, rheumatic fever or muscular rheumatism and were therefore excluded from the study. Of the remaining 118 patients, 22 had erosive arthritis, 10 had severely deforming arthritis and disorganisation of many joints (including 4 patients with typical arthritis mutilans) and 86 had a form of arthritis that was indistinguishable from that of RA.

The 22 patients with erosive arthritis met the criteria for "psoriatic arthropathy" having distal joint involvement (see X-ray) and nail changes of some digits. Their disease was relatively mild and often mistaken for gout, and they had a negative RW test. Of the 86 patients with what appeared to be RA, only 20 had a positive RW test and, in some cases, subcutaneous nodules characteristic of RA. These most likely were cases of psoriasis with coincidental RA. However, the other 66 had a negative RW test, and the age of onset was younger, fewer joints were involved and there was less disability in these psoriatic patients than that found in RA suggesting that they were not true RA.

Wright therefore proposed that all these forms of arthritis, erosive, deforming and rheumatoid-like, should be included in the term "psoriatic arthritis". This variability in disease expression probably explains why such confusion reigned in the literature for so many years regarding the association between psoriasis and rheumatoid arthritis.

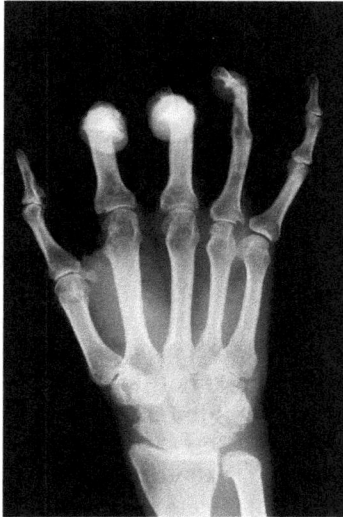

X-ray of right hand showing classical distal phalangeal joint damage in psoriatic arthritis. Wellcome Photo Library, London.

New treatments

Two new types of treatment for skin diseases became available after the war; glucocorticosteroids and folate analogues. These were probably the first drugs whose use in psoriasis was not empirical, but based upon their known mechanism of action. The anti-inflammatory effects of the glucocorticosteroid, cortisone in RA had been reported in 1949, whilst the folate analogues (aminopterin and methotrexate) were effective chemotherapy agents that inhibited cell growth.

Glucocorticosteroids

Despite its anti-inflammatory effects in RA, topical application of cortisone for the treatment of skin diseases was not found to be beneficial, despite the fact that it penetrated the skin as well as clinically effective hydrocortisone and was converted to the latter in the skin. However, the availability of synthetic derivatives of corticosteroid hormones, at the beginning of the 1950s, revolutionised the treatment of skin diseases. These

51

anti-inflammatory drugs were more potent than their natural counterparts, and, administered topically in ointments and creams, avoided the side effects experienced when the drugs were taken orally.

Adrenal cortex extracts and ACTH (corticotropin) had been used during the 1930s with variable beneficial effect in psoriasis. However, initial studies with locally applied hydrocortisone acetate in an ointment (compound F), which had been shown to be more effective than cortisone when injected into arthritic joints, had little therapeutic effect on psoriatic skin lesions. In contrast, similarly treated skin lesions of patients with atopic dermatitis were greatly improved. In 1954-5 prednisolone and fluorocortisone were introduced. Prednisolone was 4 times as powerful as cortisone, whilst the replacement of the 9-hydrogen atom by halogen fluoride in fluorocortisone resulted in a 8-fold increase in its anti-inflammatory properties. Topical preparations of fluorocortisone, although clinically superior, were soon abandoned because of their effects on electrolyte balance resulting from absorption into the systemic circulation. The additional substitution of hydroxyl or methyl groups at position 16 on the steroid molecule was subsequently found to greatly reduce the unwanted side effects induced by the fluoride atom, without significantly affecting its potentiating effect on anti-inflammatory activity. This led to the development of a wide variety of fluorinated steroids, including triamcinolone, dexamethasone and betamethasone.

Triamcinolone became available in 1958 and was administered systemically and topically in psoriasis with favourable results. In a study of 16 chronic cases of psoriasis, triamcinolone (Adcortyl tablets) was given over a period of 7-8 weeks, during which time the dose was gradually decreased[7]. Itching was relieved within 7 days, whilst clearance was observed within 3-7 weeks of commencing treatment in all but 2 of the patients. Furthermore, a third of the patients remained clear 10 weeks after the end of treatment. Minor side effects were experienced by only 2 patients in this study, and disappeared soon after completion of the course of treatment. However serious side effects such as "buffalo hump", hairy red face, decalcification of bone and hypertension, were reported with higher doses of steroids and led to the discontinuation of the use of systemic steroids in psoriasis over the next few years, except in severe cases such as erythroderma. Triamcinolone acetonide was also used locally to treat psoriasis, either by intralesional injection, or combined with other treatments such as tar, which was more effective than steroid alone.

Many more new steroids in topical formulations with the advantages of

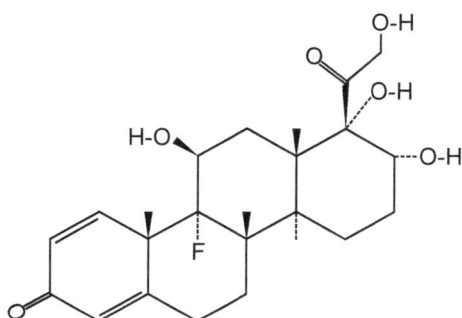

Triamcinolone

being rapidly effective, easily applied, cosmetically acceptable and stable in various vehicles were subsequently developed. However, together with increased potency came the increased likelihood of local side effects such as striae and atrophy of the skin, steroid-induced acne, purpura and glaucoma. Furthermore, systemic side effects could also be a problem (especially in children) if sufficient amounts of a potent steroid were absorbed, particularly if applied under occlusion.

Folate analogues

During the 1940s in New York, the Lederle Pharmaceutical company were testing various compounds known as anti-folates or folate analogues which inhibit the body's use of folic acid, a vitamin essential for cell growth. These compounds exert their effects by blocking the reduction of folic acid to tetrahydrofolic acid (citrovorum factor), preventing synthesis of deoxyribonucleic acid (DNA), ribonucleic acid (RNA) and proteins. The first of these anti-folates (or anti-metabolites) that showed potential as a chemotherapy drug was aminopterin, which was first reported in 1948 to produce temporary remission of acute leukaemia of children. Subsequently, in 1951 it was used experimentally to treat RA, and long-standing, extensive psoriasis with or without arthritis, inducing improvement in both skin and joints within 2 weeks after the start of treatment[8,9]. However, toxic effects such as ulceration of buccal mucosa, cramps and diarrhoea (due to inhibition of epithelial cell proliferation in the oral cavity and gastrointestinal tract), commonly accompanied the improvement in skin lesions[8]. This necessitated a rest period between

53

courses of treatment to allow the symptoms to disappear, which they usually did after a few days. In some cases citrovorum factor, which had just become available at the time, was administered to alleviate the side effects, but this lessened the therapeutic efficacy of the drug. Subsequent courses of treatment with aminopterin were sometimes combined with intramuscular or oral cortisone, which gave more complete relief of arthritic symptoms but had no additive effect on skin lesions.

Topical aminopterin in an ointment base was also tested, but was found to be ineffective in patients with psoriasis who had previously responded to the drug given orally[8].

A later study showed that normalisation of various epidermal parameters paralleled resolution of the skin lesions treated with aminopterin[10]. This was one of the first attempts made to discover the mode of action of a therapeutic treatment in psoriasis, and was made possible by knowledge of the drug's mechanism of action.

Aminopterin was replaced by its methyl derivative, amethopterin, or methotrexate as it is now known. Clinical trials showed that, like aminopterin, methotrexate was effective in causing remission in childhood leukaemia and also in the fast growing, pregnancy related cancer, choriocarcinoma, via its inhibition of the metabolism of rapidly dividing cells. Methotrexate was first used to treat psoriasis in the late 1950s, and became popular throughout the following decade. Aminopterin and methotrexate were equally effective in psoriasis and, in one study, three-quarters of the patients receiving the folic acid antagonists showed 50-100% improvement in their skin lesions that was maintained for at least 6 months[11]. However, toxicity was a major concern associated with the use of these drugs, whose side effects included modification of liver function, bone marrow depression, gastrointestinal ulcerations and bleeding, alopecia, and damage to embryonic tissue when given in high doses. In psoriasis (and RA), therapeutic effects without demonstrable toxic effects were achieved with much lower doses of methotrexate than those used in leukaemia, in which, conversely, there was a direct relationship between therapeutic and toxic effects.

Guidelines for the use of methotrexate in psoriasis and psoriatic arthritis, such as the doses to be given, the frequency of liver biopsies and the monitoring of side effects were initially suggested in the early 1970s, and were continually revised over the next decade. Furthermore, it was suggested in several studies that the development of liver damage could not be predicted by monitoring liver function tests alone. Concomitant use of alcohol, as well as increased age and body weight were identified as being significant contributors to adverse hepatic outcomes including cirrhosis. Despite three decades of study into its clinical effects, it was not until 1988 that methotrexate was approved by the U.S. Food and Drug Administration for use in adults for the treatment of immunological diseases. Furthermore, although methotrexate is commonly prescribed by rheumatologists it is still not, even now, licensed for use in psoriatic arthritis.

~ 7~

The 1960s

During the 1960s, the mechanisms underlying abnormal epidermal growth in psoriatic skin lesions became a focus of research, giving rise to the proposal that psoriasis may result from defective growth regulation. At the same time, the possibility that psoriasis may be an autoimmune or allergic condition was just beginning to be considered. The first large-scale epidemiology studies of psoriasis were performed in Scandinavia, providing further supportive evidence for a genetic basis for the disease; hydroxyurea and topical retinoic acid were introduced as new additions to the treatment armoury.

Increased epidermal turnover: defective regulation?

Although psoriasis had been recognised in the previous century as a disease of abnormal growth of epidermal cells, it wasn't until the 1960s that the mechanisms involved began to be investigated. In an early study, the location of mitoses (dividing cells) in stained sequential skin sections of psoriasis were observed and recorded on paper and in acrylic plastic models[1]. The findings demonstrated that the growth of the epidermis was caused primarily by expansion of the proliferating cell population in the lower layers of the epidermis. In a psoriatic lesion dividing cells were observed in 3 epidermal layers, compared to only one in non-involved skin. Furthermore, the length of the epidermal layers were extended more than 3-fold by enlarged dermal papillae (superficial projections of the dermis), giving an approximately 9-fold increase in the number of proliferating cells per unit length of epidermis.

Interestingly, the presence of large numbers of proliferating cells were also observed in the dermal papillae of psoriatic skin, some of which were identified as the cells lining blood vessels (endothelial cells), whilst the other cell types were not then recognised. This was probably the first report of the proliferation of lymphocytes (immune cells) in psoriatic skin lesions, a cell type whose role was to be the focus of intense research from the next decade onwards.

Increased mitotic activity in psoriatic skin was subsequently confirmed by a new approach, which combined intradermal injection of radioactive isotopes such as tritiated thymidine, with subsequent analysis by high-resolution autoradiography. Technical advances had made it possible to locate the site of isotope incorporation into cells by applying a thin film of photographic emulsion over histological slides. This was further improved by the availability of tritium-labelled isotopes, which gave a finer resolution due to the less penetrating nature of their nuclear emissions. Since thymidine is the only base incorporated exclusively into DNA, it became possible using tritiated thymidine to specifically label (black silver grains) and localise those cells in a population that were actively synthesising DNA in preparation for mitosis.

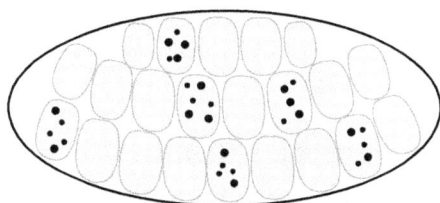

Mitotic cells labelled by autoradiography

Comparison of psoriatic and normal skin revealed that the epidermal turnover rate was significantly faster in psoriatic skin lesions, although there was some disagreement between authors as to the exact times involved[2,3]. This implied that one of the stages leading to division of an epidermal cell (the cell cycle) may be reduced in psoriasis. The location of the defect varied between studies, probably reflecting methodological differences[3,4].

In contrast to the studies carried out *in vivo*, the total cell cycle times of normal and psoriatic epidermal cells were similar in culture[5]. This resulted from a speeding up of the normal, and a lengthening of the psoriatic cell cycle times, demonstrating that epidermal cells in psoriasis are not permanently committed to abnormal proliferation. These findings were compatible with the observation that spontaneous resolution of psoriatic skin lesions occurred in a small proportion of patients, and implied that a stimulus was required to induce abnormal growth in psoriasis.

The idea that the whole skin in psoriasis was abnormal was suggested by the Koebner phenomenon (the induction of psoriatic skin lesions by trauma at any site on the body), and by the presence of disease-related changes in non-lesional skin from psoriatic patients. Thus a popular working hypothesis at this time was that the genetic defect in psoriasis was present throughout the skin and that this was manifested as the production of skin lesions in response to unknown stimuli(s). The major abnormality in psoriatic skin was widely accepted as being an increased rate of epidermal cell turnover, but the psoriatic epidermis did not appear to differ metabolically from other kinds of rapidly proliferating epidermis such as that found in wound healing. These findings led to the hypothesis, proposed by Farber and Cox in 1967, that the primary fault in psoriasis was defective control of epidermal cell proliferation[6].

Unrestrained epidermal growth was thought to be responsible for the incomplete maturation of keratinocytes in psoriasis, indicated by the lack of a granular layer, and the presence of nuclei in the stratum corneum. This proposal was consistent with the beneficial effects of current treatments at the time such as mercury, irradiation, and methotrexate, which inhibited cell proliferation, but it was less clear how glucocorticosteroids fitted into this scenario as they did not consistently suppress epithelial cell mitosis *in vivo*. However doubts were cast on the idea that incomplete cell maturation was simply a consequence of hyperproliferation by the finding that, when psoriatic lesions cleared with topical treatments, the granular layer often reformed prior to a significant reduction in the mitotic counts[7]. This was supported by the observation that a prominent granular layer is present in epidermal hyperproliferative conditions such as lamellar ichthyosis and epidermolytic hyperkeratosis.

Is psoriasis an autoimmune disease?

The recognition that humans and animals can become immunised against their own tissues and organs (auto-immunisation) led to studies of various diseases, including psoriasis, for evidence of autoreactivity. Experiments carried out in animals showed that auto-immunisation could be either cellular or antibody-mediated. However, delayed cellular responses to their own skin grafts were not observed in psoriatic patients whether the graft was from non-lesional or lesional skin. Furthermore, the injection of emulsions of full-thickness skin (normal, non-lesional or lesional psoriatic), or of their own leukocytes, into the skin of patients with psoriasis failed to induce any response [8].

The possible production of autoantibodies against skin antigens in psoriasis was investigated by two different approaches, with conflicting findings.

The first involved the use of the passive cutaneous anaphylactic (PCA) reaction, a highly sensitive method for detecting known antigen/antibody interactions. This consisted of several intradermal injections of psoriatic sera into the skin of guinea pigs, followed 6-18 hours later by the administration of a homogenate of psoriatic skin by intravenous injection. If autoantibodies to skin antigens were present in the psoriatic sera, a positive skin reaction would be observed when the injected skin antigens bound to the antibodies in the skin. Although initial studies appeared to show positive skin reactions by this procedure, these findings were discredited by the demonstration that fresh, undiluted sera alone exerted toxic effects on guinea pig skin[9]. Even when these irritant properties were reduced, administration of the skin homogenate failed to produce a positive reaction.

The second approach employed haemagglutination tests using sheep red cells that had been subjected to mild treatment with tannic acid so that they adsorbed soluble antigens onto their surface. These so-called "tanned" red cells were coated with skin antigens, obtained from the fluid of blisters induced by brief contact of skin with solid carbon dioxide. Any antibodies to skin antigens present in the tested sera bound to the red cells causing them to agglutinate. This method had been successfully used to demonstrate the production of antibodies to skin antigens in patients with second or third degree burns[8]. Although high serum antibody levels were found in psoriasis patients with extensive skin lesions (but not in corresponding patients with eczema), correlation between the level of antibodies and clinical course was found in less than half of these patients, questioning the relevance of these findings to pathogenesis.

The production of autoantibodies against skin antigens by psoriatic individuals was to be revisited a decade later using immunochemical techniques, and to lead to a new hypothesis of disease pathogenesis (see Chapter 8).

A small number of studies carried out at this time investigated the immune response in psoriasis patients, but failed to find any defects as compared to non-psoriatic controls. These included delayed hypersensitivity tests to a series of intradermally injected bacterial and fungal antigens, antibody titres to *Candida* antigens, and measurement of a local inflammatory response by the skin window technique. The latter involved collection of the fluid and cells released after abrasion of the skin, using filter paper, or a slide or coverslip. There was also no difference in the frequencies with which psoriatic patients were sensitised to contact sensitisers such as dinitrochlorobenzene; the immediate cutaneous hypersensitivity reaction to histamine was also normal.

Hydroxyurea

Methotrexate was beginning to be more widely used to treat severe psoriasis at this time, but toxic effects of the drug were a major concern. Thus new anti-metabolites were being sought that had reduced toxicity, but equal efficacy to methotrexate. Hydroxyurea was first used to treat two patients with psoriasis in 1965 with encouraging results. This drug was first synthesised nearly a century earlier, but it wasn't until 1960 that its anti-tumour activity was demonstrated in animal screening studies. Hydroxyurea inhibits DNA synthesis without significant inhibition of RNA or protein synthesis, and studies in mice have shown that it is a potent inhibitor of DNA synthesis in skin. A double-blind study of the use of hydroxyurea in psoriasis demonstrated both clinical and histopathological responses to the anti-metabolite with no adverse toxic reactions[10]. However, hydroxyurea causes (reversible) depression of the bone marrow, is teratogenic (interferes with foetal growth and development) and cannot therefore be taken during pregnancy, and can cause some impairment of renal function at high doses. Thus, although hydroxyurea is probably less toxic than methotrexate, its potentially serious side effects necessitate that it is used with caution.

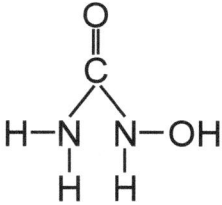

Hydroxyurea

Vitamin A (retinoic acid)

The original clinical use of vitamin A was based upon the observation that, in certain laboratory animals and in humans, vitamin A deficiency was associated with scaling of the skin, which cleared when vitamin A was added to the diet. However, vitamin A deficiency has not been found in most scaling skin diseases, and oral administration of vitamin A was rarely beneficial.

In psoriasis, topical administration of vitamin A in different forms gave variable results. Vitamin A (retinoic) acid was found to be the most potent topical vitamin A compound in psoriasis, and in other skin diseases associated with epidermal hyperproliferation[11]. Clinical improvement was seen in the majority of treated patients and was accompanied by replacement of the granular layer and a significant decrease in mitotic counts. It was considered likely that retinoic acid was beneficial in psoriasis via its effects on keratinisation rather than on mitosis, which, in mice, was stimulated by topical application of the drug at high concentrations.

Epidemiology

It had long been acknowledged that psoriasis was almost certainly an inherited disease, and several family studies had provided evidence that were consistent with this proposal. During the 1960s, the first large-scale epidemiological studies of psoriasis were carried out in the Faroe Islands[12] and in Sweden[13], involving 30,000 and 40,000 individuals, respectively, which provided further evidence for a genetic basis for the disease. These revealed significantly higher incidences of psoriasis in relatives compared to the general population, or to matched controls. The risk to first-degree relatives was estimated to be 8-23% and the prevalence of psoriasis 2-2.8% in the study populations as a whole. In the study of the disease in the Faroe Islands, 91% of patients with psoriasis had a family history, but this probably reflected the fact that the population lived in a closed community. Re-examination of the data from these studies approximately 30 years later showed its compatibility with the current concept of a polygenic model of inheritance in psoriasis.

The epidemiology of psoriasis was also studied by a questionnaire survey of 2,144 psoriatic patients from the US carried out during 1959-1968[14]. This study was unique in that data was analysed using computer processing and the standard FORTRAN programming language, the first version of which had been published about 10 years earlier. Forty questions were analysed generating 700 frequency tables, only 20 of which were selected for publication. A considerable amount of information was produced by this approach, but, as the findings were wholly dependant upon the accuracy of the participants' answers, some caution should be employed when drawing conclusions from this data.

~ 8 ~

The 1970s

The recent discovery of HLA antigens provided a new avenue of research for psoriasis during this decade. Several HLA associations were found, the strongest to a MHC Class I allele (Cw6), but the biological relevance of these findings was unknown. One proposal was that Cw6 was linked on the same chromosome to a gene predisposing to psoriasis, a view which would be supported by substantial evidence by the end of the century. These findings stimulated studies of humoral immunity in psoriasis, which revealed the deposition of various types of autoantibodies in lesional skin. In addition, the nature of the molecular defect in the skin responsible for abnormal epidermal growth became a focus of research, but there was little convincing evidence that any of the defects found were of a primary nature. This increased knowledge of the psoriatic process stimulated three new theories to explain the pathogenesis of psoriasis. Two new treatments for psoriasis, photochemotherapy, and climatotherapy at the Dead Sea, were introduced. These proved to be so successful that they remain in common use today.

HLA antigens

The observation that tissue transplants between mice of different strains were rejected, whereas those between mice of the same inbred strain were not, led to the identification of a major genetic locus which was named the Major Histocompatibility Complex or MHC. The genes in the MHC responsible for tissue rejection are very polymorphic, that is, there are many different forms or alleles in a population. The MHC genes code for cell surface glycoproteins known as major histocompatibility antigens which differ between strains of mice and which induce the production of antibodies. Antibodies, also termed immunoglobulins, bind specifically to the antigen against which they were produced; in this case, they are known as alloantibodies. In humans, alloantibodies are present in patients who have received several blood transfusions, and in women who have given birth more than once and produced antibodies against paternal alloantigens expressed by their babies *in utero*. Analysis of these

63

alloantibodies in serum enabled the major histocompatibility antigens to be defined. These were separated into two distinct classes; MHC Class I, present on nearly all cells of the body, and MHC Class II, which have a more restricted expression on cells which present foreign antigens to thymus-derived (T) lymphocytes (see below).

Serological studies of MHC Class I antigens using antisera of defined specificity began in the 1950s and were used to identify individual antigens, to determine their frequencies in populations, and to follow their inheritance in families. As the complexity of the system began to become apparent, one of the first tasks of the International Workshops set up in the mid 1960s to facilitate developments in this area was to propose a common nomenclature: Human Leukocyte Antigen (HLA). It was not until 1975 that it was realised that the HLA antigens that had been recognised thus far were derived from 2 different genes, HLA-A and HLA-B. Subsequently a third locus, HLA-C, was discovered. The HLA-C antigens were given a "w" prefix to avoid confusion with the nomenclature for complement components.

The MHC Class II antigens were discovered in the 1970s using the mixed lymphocyte culture, a technique in which lymphocytes of different individuals are cultured together. If the cells differ, they are stimulated to divide. On the other hand, a lack of response indicates a shared antigen specificity. The HLA polymorphisms detected using these cellular assays were initially called lymphocyte-defined histocompatibility antigens, which was later changed to HLA-Dw antigens. HLA polymorphisms were also detected on B cells and macrophages using antisera, and were referred to as HLA-DR (from HLA-D related) antigens; these did not always correlate exactly with those defined by cellular assays.

These developments had a significant impact, not only in the field of organ transplantation, but also for research into various inflammatory and autoimmune diseases, including psoriasis. HLA associations in psoriasis were widely studied with early reports consistently showing increased frequencies of the MHC Class I antigens, HLA-B13 and HLA-B17, particularly in patients with an earlier onset of disease[1]. Furthermore, patients expressing HLA-B17 had a high frequency of affected relatives, whilst patients expressing another Class I allele HLA-B12, which was decreased in frequency in psoriasis, had a correspondingly infrequent family history[2].

A significant association between expression of HLA-B13 and/or HLA-

B17, and streptococcal-related initiation and worsening of psoriasis was observed in some studies. Other Class I alleles such as HLA-A1, -A2 and HLA-B37 were also found to be significantly elevated in some patients. Interestingly, in a study carried out in 1970, M protein expressed in the cell wall of streptococci associated with psoriasis was shown to prevent the killing of lymphocytes by anti-sera defining several HLA-A antigens[3]. This suggested that there was a similarity in structure between the bacterial protein and HLA determinants, which could potentially lead to cross-reactivity and the development of an autoimmune response. Such a mechanism provided a possible explanation for the HLA-determined predisposition to psoriasis.

The strongest associations observed in psoriasis were for HLA-Cw6 (which was more marked in guttate than in chronic plaque psoriasis), and a Class II allele, HLA-Drw7, both of which appeared to be linked to the B locus antigens. The Cw6 and DRw7 alleles were common to psoriasis patients with or without arthritis, but patients with psoriatic arthritis also had increased frequencies of HLA-A26, HLA-B27, HLA-B38 and DRw4. Thus genetic differences as well as similarities were observed in the two populations of psoriasis patients.

Although associations with MHC Class I alleles were observed in various autoimmune and inflammatory diseases, the strongest associations were commonly with MHC Class II alleles, such as Drw4 found in RA. The strong association of a MHC Class I allele (Cw6) with psoriasis was, therefore, of particular interest.

The biological significance of the findings in psoriasis was unknown and various hypotheses were put forward, including the possibility that the HLA allele(s) was linked to a gene predisposing to psoriasis on the same chromosome. In this situation, the HLA gene could alter the expression of the pathologic gene, or, alternatively, it could act purely as a genetic marker with no functional consequences. Another suggestion was that the association with disease may not be genetically linked. In this case, the HLA antigens could cross-react with an bacterial protein, as suggested above, or interfere with membrane hormonal receptors and thus disturb epidermal cell proliferation pathways. Even now, 30 years on, the role of Cw6 in psoriasis remains unclear, although current genetic studies have provided strong evidence in support of the presence of a disease susceptibility gene close to the Cw6 gene locus (see Chapter 10).

Autoantibodies in situ

Several diseases that showed associations with HLA antigens displayed perturbations of the immune system. This was also true in psoriasis, with various studies showing autoantibody production in patients with the disease[4].

Antibodies to IgG

Antibodies against immunoglobulin (Ig)G, the major subclass of serum immunoglobulin, were detected in psoriatic sera using an absorption-elution method or by indirect immunofluorescence. These antibodies are equivalent to rheumatoid factor present in RA, but are usually of the IgG rather than IgM subclass. The immunofluorescence technique was developed in 1950 by Coons and Kaplan, and involved the use of antibodies conjugated to a fluorochrome (fluorescein isothiocyanate), which emitted light after excitation by UV light. The indirect method involved two steps; the test sera, followed by a second layer of fluorescein-conjugated antibody specific for human immunoglobulin, in this case, IgG.

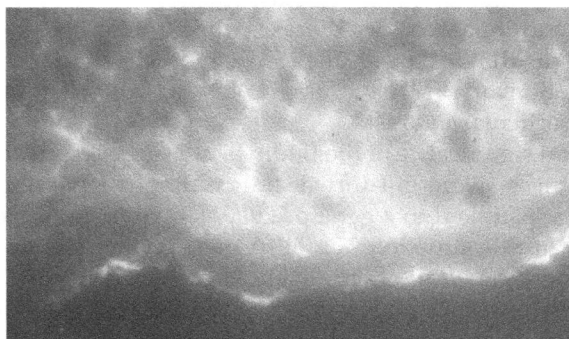

Example of indirect fluorescent staining of epidermis

These IgG anti-IgG factors, which were not detected by classical agglutination techniques, were also found on the surface of peripheral blood lymphocytes and in the epidermis of psoriatic lesions. This suggested that they might pass into the epidermis from the blood and become bound to antigen-antibody complexes. The presence of immunoglobulins and the

C3 fragment of complement in psoriatic epidermis, as described below, supported this idea.

Other autoantibodies that were detected bound to psoriatic epidermis were directed against the stratum corneum (the uppermost layer of the epidermis), or the nucleus of cells in the basal epidermal layer .

Anti-stratum corneum antibodies

Anti-stratum corneum antibodies, demonstrated by indirect immunofluorescence on normal human skin, were found in most human sera and were primarily of the IgG and IgM classes and capable of fixing complement. Complement fixation involves the activation of complement, one of the enzyme systems present in serum, followed by deposition of the activated components on nearby immune complexes, or cell membranes resulting in cell lysis.

These antibodies did not appear to bind to their corresponding antigen *in vivo* in normal individuals, whereas their presence was demonstrated using the direct immunofluorescence technique (anti-human IgG conjugate alone) in psoriatic scale. The staining was widespread and consistent in fully developed active psoriatic lesions, but was absent from non-lesional psoriatic skin. In addition, complement components C3 and/or C4 were also demonstrated in most cases in a comparable pattern in the stratum corneum. Deposits of immunoglobulins, probably anti-stratum corneum antibodies, and complement were also found in some other skin conditions such as eczema, but the staining pattern was different compared to psoriatic skin and the deposits only transiently present.

These observations led to a new hypothesis proposed by Beutner et al[5] to explain the pathogenesis of psoriasis that implicated polymorphonuclear leukocytes in the development of skin lesions. It was proposed that the release of proteolytic enzymes by these inflammatory cells, which entered the skin in response to trauma or infection, could convert the normally inaccessible stratum corneum antigen into a reactive form. The dilation of blood vessels accompanying this reaction would allow the anti-stratum corneum antibodies to enter the epidermis and bind, thus triggering the disease process. The ensuing complement fixation and production of chemotactic complement components would then attract more polymorphonuclear leukocytes into the psoriatic stratum corneum, thus maintaining the pathological cycle. However, the increased epidermal growth rate is not adequately explained by this hypothesis, as the polymorphonuclear leukocytes are situated in the stratum corneum layers, far from the proliferating basal keratinocytes. In addition, it raises the question as to why trauma would not lead to the formation of a psoriatic lesion in a normal individual. The absence of anti-stratum corneum antibodies in the early pre-pinpoint skin lesion, and the influx of polymorphonuclear leukocytes subsequent to that of lymphocytes suggest that this process cannot trigger psoriasis, but does not exclude the possibility of its involvement in the maintenance of a psoriatic lesion.

Anti-nuclear antibodies

The other type of autoantibodies reported in psoriatic skin lesions were anti-nuclear antibodies, which were demonstrated bound to nuclei retained in the stratum corneum. They were not restricted to any one immunoglobulin subclass, were also present on lymphoid cells and polymorphonuclear cells in the dermal infiltrate and Munro abscesses, respectively, but were not detected in sera.

Antibodies predominately reactive with basal cell nuclei have also been demonstrated on the membranes of circulating lymphoid cells and polymorphonuclear cells in psoriatic patients. These antibodies were not present in healthy controls, did not fix complement and only reacted with nuclei of epidermal cells in non-lesional skin of psoriatic individuals. These observations led to a further hypothesis for psoriasis, proposed by Cormane and colleagues[6], which suggested that anti-basal cell nuclear antibodies might detach from locally recruited inflammatory cells and bind to receptors on basal cell membranes, inducing a shift of cells from the resting phase into the proliferating pool. Alternatively, such antibodies could conceivably have a regulatory rather than stimulatory role.

The reports of increased levels of serum (and salivary) IgA and IgE in psoriasis, together with the presence of autoantibodies in psoriatic skin, suggested a defect in the regulation of the immune response. It had been discovered a few years previously that IgA and IgE production by B cells was dependent upon cooperation with thymus-derived (T) lymphocytes. Thus, the first investigations of T lymphocytes in psoriasis began during the 1970s, with mixed results. Numbers of T cells were determined using E-rosette tests. These tests were based upon the observation that human T cells have receptors for sheep erythrocytes (E) or red cells, forming rosettes which can then be counted or isolated for functional studies. A significant decrease in T cell numbers was shown in some studies, whilst in others, no T cell defect was found. These discrepancies may be related to the activity of the skin lesions, and therefore secondary to the disease process.

Stimulation of T cell proliferation using the plant lectin, concanavalin A, showed a decreased response by psoriatic lymphocytes, which led to the speculation that there may be a selective deficiency of a suppressor T cell subpopulation in psoriasis, which would be consistent with autoantibody production[7].

The first studies of the nature of the mononuclear cell infiltrate in psoriatic skin lesions were also performed during this period; these showed that the majority of infiltrating cells were T lymphocytes and macrophages [8,9].

Molecular nature of skin defect

Based upon the premise that the primary genetic defect in psoriasis is located in the skin, the possible molecular nature of such a defect began to be investigated. Candidates considered for the role included cyclic nucleotides, polyamines, and arachidonic acid and its metabolites[10].

Cyclic nucleotides

In 1971, Voorhees and Duell[11] first proposed that a defective cyclic adenosine monophosphate (cAMP) cascade might trigger the onset of psoriasis, and/or allow the disease process to be maintained. The hypothesis was based upon the observation that cAMP could induce breakdown of glycogens and decrease proliferation, whilst increasing differentiation. Decreased cAMP levels would thus explain three characteristics of psoriatic epidermis; increased proliferation, increased epidermal glycogen content, and decreased terminal differentiation. The statistically significantly decreases in cAMP levels in lesional compared to non-lesional psoriatic epidermis reported by the same group in initial studies, were not, however, confirmed in studies performed by other workers using different cAMP assay methods, or by the same group using a more sensitive and specific assay. Thus it seemed likely that the steady-state level of cAMP was not altered in psoriatic epidermis.

However, there was some evidence that the inducibility of cAMP levels may be altered. Hormone-like molecules such as beta catecholamines, adenosine, histamine, prostaglandins of the E series (see below) and cholera toxin can increase intracellular cAMP levels via interaction with cell surface receptors coupled to the enzyme adenylate cyclase. In psoriatic lesions, the ability of beta and prostaglandin receptors to generate cAMP was reduced. Furthermore cAMP phosphodiesterase, an enzyme that degrades cAMP, was found to be twice as active in psoriatic epidermis, which could modify cAMP levels.

In contrast, cyclic guanosine monophosphate (cGMP) levels were increased in psoriatic epidermis, resulting in a decreased cAMP/cGMP ratio. This was partly due to stimulation of cGMP synthesis by the polyunsaturated fatty acid, arachidonic acid and its metabolite, 12-hydroxy-eicosatetraenoic acid , and partly to inhibition of the adenylate cyclase enzyme leading to reduced cAMP synthesis (see below). The significance of increased cGMP levels in the epidermis to the psoriatic process was, however, unknown.

There is some support for a role for a defective cAMP system in the pathogenesis of psoriasis. For example it has been observed that lithium, a known inhibitor of adenyl cyclase, induces and exacerbates psoriasis. Whether this drug directly affects the epidermis or acts via the immune system to induce clinical expression has not been established. Beta receptor-blocking agents such as practolol and propranolol exacerbate pre-existing psoriasis and can even induce the first expression of plaque-type or pustular psoriasis. Furthermore, intradermal injection of propranolol increases the number of proliferating cells in psoriatic epidermis more than in normal skin. Conversely, agents that inhibit the enzyme breakdown of cAMP, such as papaverine, have been reported to improve psoriasis. However, these drugs have several known mechanisms of action that could account for their effects, including, in the case of propranolol, effects on some immune functions. Overall, the findings were consistent with the possibility that a defective cAMP pathway could contribute to the abnormal growth of the epidermis in psoriasis, but there was little convincing evidence that a defect of this kind was of a primary nature.

Polyamines

Polyamines are low molecular weight amines that are essential to cell proliferation. They are increased in actively proliferating cells, and can stimulate RNA and protein synthesis *in vivo*. Not surprisingly, therefore, the polyamines, putrescine and spermidine, and their biosynthetic enzyme ornithine decarboxylase (ODC), were all reported to be elevated in psoriatic skin relative to normal or non-lesional skin. In certain tissues,

ODC, and therefore polyamine formation is regulated by cAMP. An inability to inhibit ODC activity due to a defective cAMP cascade could explain the raised polyamine levels in psoriatic epidermis. In any event, although these abnormalities may affect the regulation of epidermal growth, it is unlikely that increased polyamine levels represent a primary defect in psoriatic skin, as they are common to several other situations in which epidermal hyperproliferation occurs.

Arachidonic acid and its metabolites

Arachidonic acid (AA) is stored with other polyunsaturated fatty acids in cell membranes where it is bound as phospholipid. Once released, AA is converted via two different pathways into several different biologically active compounds. One pathway involves a cyclic oxygenase, giving rise to 20-carbon, fatty acids known as prostaglandins (PGs). The other produces hydroxy-eicosatetraenoic acids (HETE's) and leukotrienes, via the action of lipoxygenases.

Several studies indicated that AA metabolism was misregulated in psoriasis. Thus extremely high levels of free AA and 12-HETE, together with a more modest elevation of PGE_2 and $PGF_{2\alpha}$ levels were reported, suggesting that prostaglandin biosynthesis may be inhibited in psoriatic epidermis. This was postulated to divert increased amounts of free AA to the lipoxygenase system and the production of leukotrienes. Leukotrienes were suspected to play an important role in the pathogenesis of psoriasis, because some of the features characteristic of psoriasis can be explained, at least in part, by their action. Leukotrienes and HETEs are important mediators of inflammation. Furthermore, leukotriene B_4 is an extremely potent chemotactic agent for polymorphonuclear leukocytes, and, in addition, stimulates epidermal cell proliferation *in vitro*[12].

Treatment of psoriasis with agents that selectively modulated the production of AA-derived products supported a role for leukotrienes in the psoriatic process. For example, application of indomethacin, a cyclooxygenase inhibitor, to psoriatic plaques increased disease activity[13], presumably by further increasing the diversion of free AA into the lipoxygenase system. Conversely, the 5-lipoxygenase inhibitor benoxaprofen markedly improved psoriasis[14]. Its use was later discontinued because of hepatotoxic and phototoxic side-effects.

Although leukotrienes are probably involved in the disease process, advancements made in the years leading up to the end of the 20th century would show that products made by T lymphocytes (cytokines) would play a much more important role in the immunopathogenesis of psoriasis.

Guilhou's Hypothesis

In an attempt to encompass all the new information that had been generated in relation to psoriasis during this period, Guilhou et al[15] proposed a pathogenic chain of events consisting of six steps. The steps constituting the latter stages of the pathway (efferent way) were membrane abnormalities (step 3), leading to cyclic nucleotide and prostaglandin imbalance (step 2), which in turn resulted in increased epidermal proliferation (step 1). The steps making up the initial stages which resulted in membrane alterations (afferent way) were less defined, but included immunological factors such as the presence of autoantibodies bound to psoriatic epidermis (step 4), which could result from a lack of T cell regulation (step 5), which in turn may be caused by genetic and/or viral factors (step 6).

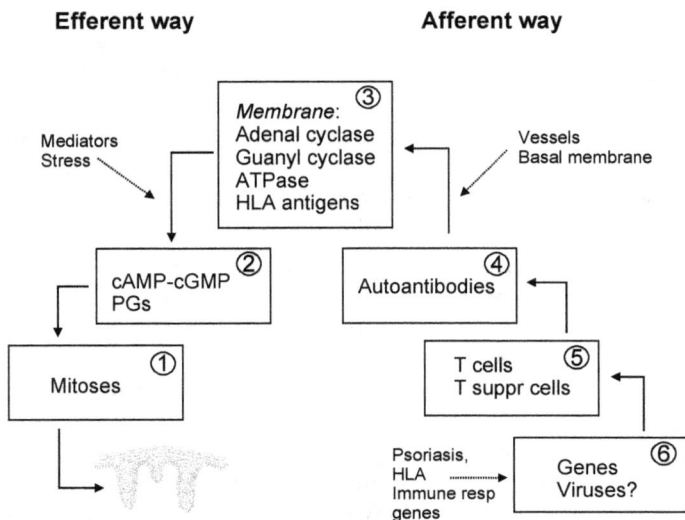

Efferent way   **Afferent way**

Mediators
Stress

Membrane: ③
Adenal cyclase
Guanyl cyclase
ATPase
HLA antigens

Vessels
Basal membrane

cAMP-cGMP ②
PGs

Autoantibodies ④

Mitoses ①

T cells ⑤
T suppr cells

Psoriasis,
HLA
Immune resp
genes

Genes ⑥
Viruses?

Guilhou's six-step hypothesis for psoriasis.

Photochemotherapy

The first use of the administration of plant extracts, followed by sun exposure (photochemotherapy) in the treatment of skin disease was by the Hindus in about 1400 BC. In 1947, the active ingredients in these plant extracts were isolated, 8-methoxypsoralen (8-MOP) and 5-methoxypsoralen (5-MOP), and used in combination with sun exposure to treat patients with vitiligo. After it had been determined that long wavelength ultraviolet radiation (320-400 nm; UVA) was the most efficient for activating 8-MOP, artificial sources of UVA were developed. These UVA tubes were used in a total-body-irradiation cabin with topical 8-MOP, initially to treat vitiligo, and then subsequently psoriasis. The results from these early studies were, however, restricted by the low output of the UV lamps at the time. In the USA in 1974, Parrish reported the use of a new type of a high intensity UVA tube in combination with oral 8-MOP for the treatment of psoriasis[16]. Soon after, a cooperative clinical trial was set up, which was one of the first and largest prospective follow-up studies of a new medical technology. This highly effective procedure became known as PUVA (psoralens + UVA), and was to revolutionise the treatment of

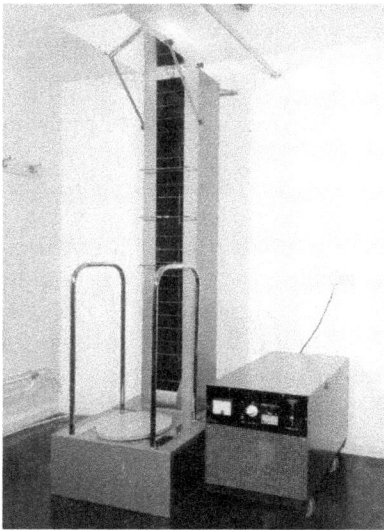

The PUVA unit used at the Kent and Canterbury Hospital in the 1970s. Courtesy of Prof. B. Diffey, University of Newcastle.

psoriasis.

In the UK, the first PUVA units were developed by medical physicists at the Ninewells Hospital, Dundee, and at the Kent and Canterbury Hospital[17]. In the latter case, use of the PUVA unit involved rotation of the patient at 3 revolutions per minute in front of the UV source. This design did not, however, catch on! This was followed by the manufacture of the first whole-body commercial PUVA unit in the UK.

The mechanism of action of PUVA in psoriasis was believed, at this time, to be a decrease in cell proliferation as a result of the formation of 8-MOP-DNA photoadducts. However, it was established some 20 years later that keratinocytes were highly resistant to the effects of PUVA therapy, and that the more sensitive T lymphocytes residing in the epidermis were more likely to be affected.

PUVA went on to become one of the mainstays of psoriasis therapy, although concerns about the development of skin cancers were to modify its use.

Dead Sea therapy (Climatotherapy)

The use of balneotherapy (immersion of patients in mineral water baths or pools) and spa therapy as accompaniments to psoriasis treatment first emerged during the 19th century. Since that time, three unique locations for balneotherapy have become established; the Blue Lagoon in Iceland, the Kangal hot spring in Turkey, and, most importantly, the Dead Sea in Israel.

The healing properties of the Dead Sea (Sea of Salt in Hebrew) were recognised as early as the second century by Galen who described "the potency of this medicine (asphalt produced in the Dead Sea) consists in its drying and next its healing capabilities; it is indeed appropriate that people use it for closing bleeding wounds"[18]. Further evidence that Dead Sea water was used for healing was documented during the 3rd to 6th centuries in the Talmud, a fundamental code of civil and ecclesiastic law compiled by Jewish sages[19]. During the 18th century, geographers and scientists began renewed exploration of the area, and water from the Dead Sea was chemically analysed. Dostrovsky and coworkers published the first preliminary report of the beneficial effects of exposure to the Dead Sea on psoriasis in 1959[20], followed by numerous reports during the 1970's which confirmed the ameliorative properties of the Dead Sea environment in large numbers of patients. More than 80% of the psoriasis patients treated

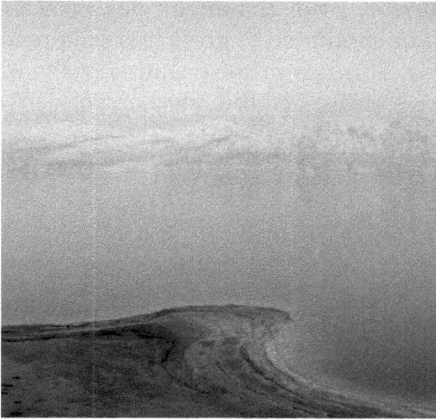

The Dead Sea: photograph taken by David Shankbone.

with daily exposure to solar UV light and regular bathing in the Dead Sea (climatotherapy) had either complete or nearly complete clearance of their skin lesions. Furthermore, patients with psoriatic arthritis also showed significant improvement in their symptoms. These beneficial effects were attributed to several factors relating to the location and characteristics of the Dead Sea.

Firstly, the Dead Sea is the lowest and most saline lake on earth, being 400m below sea level with an approximately 30% salt content. The salts (magnesium, calcium, potassium and bromine) present in the lake water, which are used in the production of various health products, contribute to the resolution of skin lesions. Mud packs and sulphur baths may also be included in the treatment regime.

Secondly, UV light is attenuated by traversing an extra 400m of atmosphere and a haze of water vapour and aerosols overhanging the lake. This changes the spectral balance, affecting UVB more than UVA, allowing longer exposure times. Thus the well known beneficial effects of UV light can be experienced with a reduced risk of burning.

Furthermore, psychological benefits are attributed to the social nature of the treatment regime. Fellow patients stay in the same hotels and share experiences, whilst the general success of the treatment generates a more optimistic outlook to living with the disease.

The success of the Dead Sea treatment, regardless of the extent of skin involvement or nature of prior treatment, has meant that thousands of psoriasis patients have continued to go to this unique location every year up to the present day. This is a prime example of the use of an empirical approach to treat psoriasis, as the mechanisms involved were, and essentially still are, unknown.

~ 9~

The 1980s

During the 1980s, the development of monoclonal antibodies led to the identification of subpopulations of cells in skin lesions. This was the beginning of a new era in which T cells and their products were to take centre stage in psoriasis research. As a direct result, the immunosuppressive drug cyclosporin, which targets activated T cells, began to be used to treat psoriasis. This marked a change from therapies used empirically to those whose use was evidence-based. Vitamin D analogues, the first oral retinoid and narrowband UVB irradiation were also introduced into the psoriasis treatment armoury. The ability of keratinocytes in psoriatic skin to produce various types of immune mediators was demonstrated, and the first mouse models for psoriasis were developed which enabled the location of the defect leading to abnormal epidermal growth to be investigated.

T cell subpopulations in skin lesions

Prior to 1980, T lymphocytes in peripheral blood and tissues were investigated using methods such as enzyme cytochemical staining, sheep red blood cell rosetting or immuno-staining with polyclonal (non-specific) antibodies against T cells. As a result of the development of monoclonal antibody hybridoma technology by Kohler and Milstein in 1975[1] it became possible, for the first time, to identify subpopulations of immune cells using highly specific probes for surface markers. Monoclonal antibodies against T cell antigens were produced by taking spleen cells from a mouse immunised with human T cells and fusing them with myeloma (plasma cell tumour) cell lines. This was followed by repeated subculture and dilution until single clones of antibody-secreting cells were established. Using monoclonal antibodies specific for the markers CD4 and CD8, T lymphocytes can be subdivided into two functional groups. T cells expressing CD4 antigen act as helper T cells that assist B cells to produce antibodies, whilst CD8[+] T cells kill infected cells and suppress responses by T and B cells.

The availability of these new monoclonal antibodies allowed T cell subpopulations, and Langerhans cells (dendritic-shaped cells that can present antigen to T cells) to be studied in skin lesions of psoriasis[2-4].

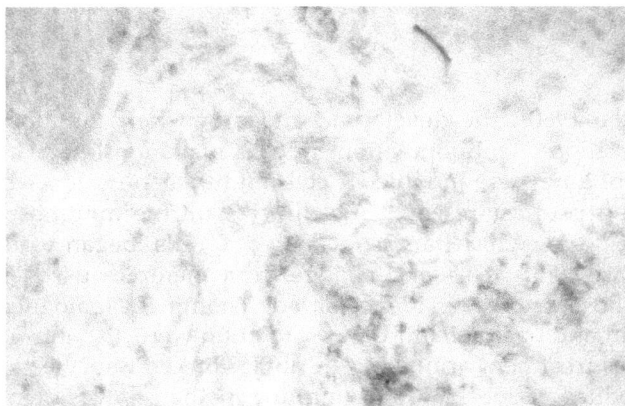

T cells stained by monoclonal antibodies in psoriatic skin.

Most of the T cells were observed in the dermis; CD4[+] T cells exceeded CD8[+] T cells by approximately 2:1, and the majority of the activated T cells were CD4[+]. However, the appearance of a clinical lesion was associated with the presence of a small number of activated CD4[+] T cells in the epidermal layer, rather than by detectable changes in the numbers of T cells in the dermis[4]. Conversely, the clearing of skin lesions coincided with increased numbers of activated CD8[+] T cells in the epidermis. Langerhans cells were observed in close proximity to T cells in the epidermis suggesting that they were interacting to generate an immune response[4]. These observations led to the suggestion that T cells may be essential participants of the psoriatic disease process.

T cell Hypothesis

The presentation of a specific antigen (by an antigen-presenting cell) to CD4[+] T cells that recognise that antigen results in their activation and the subsequent production of cytokines (previously known as lymphokines), soluble proteins which act as chemical communicators between cells. Cytokines bind to specific receptors on the surface of target cells, which are linked to intracellular signalling pathways. This results in stimulatory effects on the function of the target cells, which can be one of many different cell types, including epidermal keratinocytes. This formed the basis for a new hypothesis for psoriasis by Valdimarsson and colleagues, published in 1986, which proposed that epidermal growth was induced by a putative epidermal proliferation factor (EPF) released by activated CD4⁺ T cells within the epidermal layer[5]. Stimulation of epidermal growth would, in turn, induce production of a novel factor called epidermal thymocyte-activating factor (ETAF) released by keratinocytes[6]. This recently discovered factor was almost certainly the same as Interleukin-1 (see below), a cytokine that induces inflammation via a wide range of biological activities on many different target cells, and the first of more than 20 different interleukins that would be identified over the next 25 years. ETAF attracts T lymphocytes and, it was hypothesised, could cause these cells to migrate from the dermis into the epidermis creating a cycle of events that would maintain the psoriatic process.

T cell activators

The nature of the antigen(s) that activates T lymphocytes in psoriasis was unknown, and, 20 years on, has remained elusive. Streptococcal infections had been associated with psoriasis for approximately three decades (see Chapter 6), implicating bacterial antigens as T cell stimulators. Furthermore reaction against self-antigens as a result of streptococcal infection was postulated when it was observed that monoclonal antibodies against streptococcal antigens cross-reacted with the epidermis of skin[7]. Virus-like particles were reported in psoriasis patients in one study[8]; in addition, it was observed that patients with acquired immunodeficiency syndrome (AIDS) and psoriasis experienced worsening of their skin disease, suggesting that viral antigens may activate T cells in some patients[9].

Cytokines in skin lesions

Evidence to support an on-going immune response in psoriatic skin lesions was the demonstration that interferon-gamma (IFN-γ), a product of activated T lymphocytes, was present in the serum and fluid from suction-induced blisters of psoriasis patients[10]. This cytokine exerts a variety of functional effects on different cell types, including epidermal keratinocytes. Of relevance to the psoriatic process is its ability to influence

79

the trafficking of T lymphocytes into the epidermis via the upregulation of T cell-binding molecules on the surface of keratinocytes[11]. In addition, IFN-γ inhibits the growth of keratinocytes from normal skin. Interestingly, keratinocytes from psoriatic lesions were shown to be less susceptible than normal keratinocytes, which, it was suggested, could contribute to the increased epidermal growth and impaired differentiation in psoriasis[12]. The proposal that keratinocytes from psoriatic skin respond abnormally to IFN-γ was supported by *in vivo* studies. Intradermal injection of IFN-γ failed to inhibit DNA synthesis as measured by autoradiography[13], whilst systemic administration of the cytokine either had no clinical effect or only slightly improved the condition of some of the treated patients.

Other types of cytokines produced by keratinocytes were also demonstrated in psoriatic skin lesions; interleukins, transforming growth factors and tumour necrosis factor (TNF)-α.

In contrast to interleukin-1, which appeared to be reduced, two other cytokines, IL-6 and IL-8 were increased in psoriatic epidermis. Both IL-6, a major mediator of the host response to injury and infection, and IL-8, a potent T cell and polymorphonuclear leukocyte chemoattractant, stimulated keratinocyte growth.

Transforming growth factor (TGF)-α, which is produced by and required for the growth of epithelial cells, is also overexpressed in psoriatic epidermis, accompanied by increased expression of its receptor. It has been suggested that the numerous biochemical alterations detected in psoriatic skin during the previous decade could be accounted for, in part, by chronic receptor activation by TGF-α[14]. TGF-α may also contribute to the marked development of capillary blood vessels observed in psoriatic dermis.

Unlike these cytokines, TNF-α exerts an inhibitory effect on keratinocyte proliferation, but may contribute indirectly to epidermal growth in psoriasis by its ability to induce IL-8 and TGF-α production. Biological therapies that block TNF-α activity are currently proving to be clinically effective in patients with moderate to severe psoriasis, supporting an important role for the cytokine in the disease process (see Chapter 11).

An inherent defect of epidermal cell growth?

Unlike some other skin diseases, animals do not suffer from psoriasis, a factor that hampered progress in the understanding of the mechanisms involved in the disease process. The first attempts to develop an animal model for psoriasis were made in the early 1980s using nude mice, so called because they lack hair. These mice are born without a thymus, and therefore lack T cell function (or so it was assumed) and are unable to reject grafts of foreign tissue. Lesional and non-lesional skin from psoriasis patients, and normal skin were transplanted onto the backs of nude mice and epidermal proliferation rates were compared[15]. Before

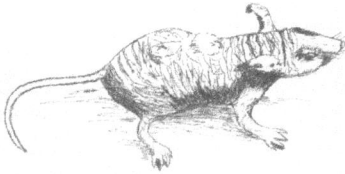

transplantation, both lesional and, to a lesser degree, non-lesional psoriatic skin showed significantly increased DNA synthesis of the epidermis, consistent with observations first made many years previously. However, 6 weeks after transplantation, the DNA synthesis in lesional skin had moderately decreased and in non-lesional skin had increased so that their proliferative activity was equally elevated as compared to normal skin, which had remained unchanged.

Nude mouse transplanted with human skin.
Illustration by Betty Baker.

A second study using nude mice reported preservation of certain immunological identities of grafted psoriatic skin, but other features such as a lack of granular layer were not maintained[16].

These observations suggested that there was an inherent defect of epidermal cell growth in patients with psoriasis, a hypothesis first put forward in 1930 by Samberger, but that host cellular and/or non-cellular factors (which were absent from the nude mouse model) modulated expression of the disease. The suitability of the nude mouse model for the study of psoriasis pathogenesis was called into question a few years later, however, when it was shown that, not only did human lymphocytes disappear from psoriatic skin transplanted onto nude mice within 48 hours, but that they were replaced by mouse T cells that may have contributed to the skin changes observed[17].

A dermal defect?

The involvement of the dermis in the stimulation of epidermal cell growth in psoriasis was also investigated during this period. One approach involved taking samples of psoriatic and normal skin, separating the epidermis from dermis, and then recombining the two layers from the different samples in various combinations before transplanting the recombinants onto nude mice[18]. Only when psoriatic epidermis was recombined with psoriatic dermis was an increased labelling index of the same magnitude as that of unseparated skin observed, suggesting that both skin compartments were necessary for abnormal epidermal cell growth.

Using a skin equivalent model, dermal fibroblasts (cells that synthesise components of connective tissue including collagen) were implicated as inducers of abnormal keratinocyte growth, whilst a specific defect of epidermal cells was excluded[19]. The skin model consisted of a small full-thickness punch biopsy inserted into a dermal equivalent, produced by the contraction of a collagen gel by dermal fibroblasts that had been grown as monolayer cultures on plastic. When the dermal equivalent was prepared from psoriatic fibroblasts, hyperproliferation of both normal and non-lesional psoriatic keratinocytes was observed suggesting that the defect was specific for psoriatic fibroblasts. However, although the evidence supported an interaction between the two skin cell types, the idea that fibroblasts were driving epidermal growth in psoriasis fell out of favour, as the role of T cells dominated psoriasis research over the next decade.

The possibility that a primary defect was located in the dermal vasculature had long been debated. However, the findings of a study examining the effects of treatment with PUVA or the Goeckerman regime on the capillaries in psoriatic skin lesions provided further support for an epidermal rather than microvascular defect[20]. The investigators carrying out the study had previously shown that arterial and venous capillaries could be differentiated by their ultrastructural features. Furthermore, in contrast to normal skin in which the capillary loops were arterial, those in psoriatic skin were of the venous type. In patients who responded to treatment, the capillaries reverted from venous to arterial type and the histological features of psoriasis disappeared, but the labelling index of the epidermal cells remained elevated suggesting that the role of the microvasculature in psoriasis is unlikely to be of a primary nature.

Evidence-based treatment: Cyclosporin

The growing possibility that T cells were responsible for the induction of epidermal cell growth in psoriasis led to the prediction that the fungal metabolite and immunosuppressive agent cyclosporin should be effective in resolving skin lesions. This was based upon the drug's known selective inhibitory effects on cytokine production by CD4+ T cells. This is probably one of the first drugs whose use in psoriasis was based upon its likely mechanism of action, which was made possible by increased knowledge of the immunopathogenic mechanisms underlying the disease. Furthermore, its' successful use in psoriasis would, in turn, provide supportive evidence for the T cell-based hypothesis. In fact, cyclosporin had already been shown, by chance, to be of benefit in psoriasis in a study in 1979 in which patients with arthritis were treated[21]. Four of the patients suffered from psoriatic arthritis, and it was observed that, not only did their arthritis improve, but also their accompanying skin lesions cleared in a matter of days. This observation was subsequently confirmed in initial trials of the drug in psoriasis patients in the UK, USA and Germany[22-24], which eventually led to its general use for severe, recalcitrant psoriasis. The initial enthusiasm for this new approach to the treatment of psoriasis has, however, been tempered over time by its dose-related side-effects, particularly nephrotoxicity and hypertension, which has restricted its use.

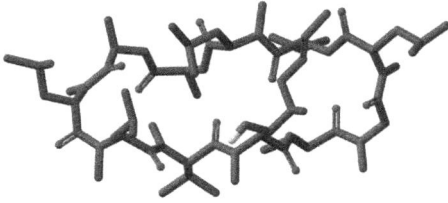

Stick model of cyclosporin by Ben Mills, 2008

Clearing of psoriasis by treatment with cyclosporin was accompanied by a decrease in CD4+ and CD8+ T cells in lesional skin[25], whilst a direct inhibitory action on epidermal keratinocytes was excluded. Similarly, decreases in skin T cells were also observed in skin lesions treated with topical steroids, psoralens plus UVA light (PUVA) or dithranol, treatments which continued to be (and still are) in current use[26,27]. The rate of disappearance of T cells from the epidermis correlated with the rate of resolution in individual patients, and in PUVA-treated patients, the depletion of epidermal T cells preceded the onset of clinical improvement.

These observations provided further supportive evidence for a role for T cells in psoriasis.

Etretinate – the first oral retinoid

During the 1960s, topical retinoic (vitamin A) acid had been used to treat psoriasis. The drug company Roche subsequently synthesized many hundreds of retinal analogues, resulting in the synthesis of etretinate in the 1970s. During the following decade, etretinate (brand name Tigason) was administered orally to patients with severe, recalcitrant or generalised pustular psoriasis, but, because of its attendant toxic side-effects, was not suitable for patients with minimal skin involvement. In order to reduce dosages, and therefore adverse toxic effects, and to improve therapeutic outcome, etretinate was also used in combination with other treatment modalities such as PUVA, corticosteroids, dithranol and methotrexate. Etretinate reduced epidermal cell growth in both lesional and non-lesional skin of psoriatic patients, but its exact mode of action was unknown. Levels of polyamines, which are involved in the regulation of cell proliferation and are increased in psoriatic skin (see Chapter 8), were decreased in the skin of etretinate-treated individuals prior to clinical improvement[28.] Furthermore, etretinate reduced ornithine decarboxylase, the enzyme necessary for polyamine synthesis[29], implicating this as the primary target of the drug's action.

The free acid derivative of etretinate (acitretin or etretin), with the advantage of a shorter half-life of elimination than etretinate, also proved to be effective in psoriasis and other diseases of keratinisation, but signs and symptoms of hypervitaminosis A were observed in some patients treated with the drug.

Vitamin D analogues

In the 1930s, vitamin D had proved to have some beneficial effects in psoriasis when administered orally. However, the hypercalcaemic side effects associated with vitamin D therapy led to its discontinuation in the 1940s. Approximately 50 years later, the beneficial effects of the vitamin in psoriasis were "rediscovered" by Japanese researchers in a patient treated with a vitamin D_3 analogue for osteoporosis, who experienced a dramatic clearing of psoriatic lesions[30]. The efficacy was attributed to its metabolite, calcitriol, which was the first of a new generation of topical vitamin D_3 analogues to be used for treatment of mild to moderate plaque psoriasis. Calcipotriol was the most extensively studied of these, and was shown to be slightly more efficacious than the topical steroid, betamethasone 17-

valerate, or dithranol. These drugs were known to modulate epidermal growth and differentiation, suggesting their mode of action in psoriasis, but later a variety of effects on cells of the immune system were also demonstrated.

Narrowband UVB

Narrow band (311nm) UVB treatment was first introduced at the end of the decade, in an attempt to reduce the incidence of burning and potential risk of carcinogenesis associated with conventional broadband (280-350nm) UVB. An experimental fluorescent lamp, the Philips TL-01, was developed which produced a peak narrow band emission at 311nm, thus excluding the non-therapeutic lower wavelengths of 290 nm and below, which were believed to contribute to UVB-induced carcinogenic effects. Preliminary studies comparing the new lamp with that of the broadband TL 40W/12 lamp demonstrated effective clearing of psoriasis with the advantages of increased duration of remission and significantly reduced incidences of burning[31]. In addition, because the number of treatments per week could be increased, resolution of psoriatic lesions was faster than with conventional UVB treatment. Confirmation of these findings in further studies ensured that narrowband UVB irradiation subsequently became a well established and widely used treatment for psoriasis, whose major mechanism of action was probably via its suppression of immune responses.

~ 10~

The 1990s

As one might expect, the greatest advances in our understanding of psoriasis have taken place during the latter part of the 20th century, accompanying the rapid pace of progress in new technology. Several observations led to the now widely accepted view that psoriasis is an immunological disease mediated by T cells. Consequently, research was focused on the characteristics of the T cells in skin lesions, including the nature of their antigen receptors and the cytokines they produce. The response to streptococcal antigens by T cells in psoriasis was also investigated, in an attempt to explain the long recognised association of streptococcal infections with the disease. As the decade came to an end, novel biological therapies began to be developed and tested, and lasers, the immunosuppressive drug, tacrolimus, and topical ascomycins and retinoids were introduced to treat psoriasis. At the same time, the search for the identity of the psoriasis genes began, made possible by the technological advances that accompanied the progress of the Human Genome Project.

Psoriasis is a T cell-mediated disease

During the 1980s, it had been demonstrated that resolution of chronic psoriasis during treatment with topical steroids, PUVA, dithranol or cyclosporin was accompanied by depletion of T cells from lesional skin, suggesting that T cells were essential to the psoriatic disease process. Subsequently, tacrolimus (FK506), another immunosuppressive drug that, in common with cyclosporin, was developed for use in organ transplantation and primarily targets T cells, was also found to be beneficial in psoriasis accompanied by a rapid disappearance of the inflammatory infiltrate. Effects on antigen-presenting cells may have also contributed to the efficacy of some of the treatments, but direct effects on epidermal cells were minimal or absent.

Various observations made during the 1990s have lent support to the T cell hypothesis, such that it is now widely accepted throughout the psoriasis research community (reviewed in Ref 1).

One study showed rapid clinical improvement in a small group of patients after intravenous administration of monoclonal antibodies directed against the CD4 molecule, expressed by the majority of activated T cells in the dermis of psoriatic skin lesions. In another study activated T cells were targeted using a fusion protein, denileukin diftitox (otherwise known as Ontak), which consists of diphtheria toxin linked to the T cell growth factor, interleukin (IL)-2[2]. Denileukin diftitox binds to activated T cells because they express the receptor for IL-2; the toxin is then taken into the cell where it induces cell death. As keratinocytes in psoriatic skin lesions lack IL-2 receptors, they are unaffected by the toxin. Correlation between the extent of the selective depletion of activated T cells in psoriatic skin lesions by denileukin diftitox and the clinical response was demonstrated, supporting a role for T cells in the disease process.

Additional evidence came from the development of a new mouse model for psoriasis consisting of Severe Combined Immunodeficient (SCID) mice, which are genetically incapable of producing either T or B cells, transplanted with non-lesional psoriatic skin[3]. When the transplanted skin was injected with pre-activated blood-derived lymphocytes and antigen-presenting cells from the same individual (autologous), conversion into a psoriatic plaque was consistently observed. However, if the same experiment was carried out with normal skin and autologous immunocytes, no psoriatic conversion took place. Using this model, it was subsequently shown that CD4[+] T cells, but not CD8[+] T cells, induced the change to psoriatic phenotype, providing further support for a pivotal role for CD4[+] T cells in the disease process[4]. This was consistent with the observation that psoriasis could be transferred by allogeneic (genetically non-identical) bone-marrow transplantation to individuals with no previous history of the disease, or conversely cleared by bone-marrow tranplantations from non-psoriatic individuals, implicating marrow-derived lymphocytes in psoriatic pathogenesis.

The demonstration that products secreted by T cells cultured from psoriasis skin lesions promoted keratinocyte growth provided a possible mechanism for the role of T cells in psoriasis. One of the cytokines involved was IFN-γ, but further cytokines were implicated but remained unidentified.

Th1 cytokines

The subdivision of CD4⁺ T cells into two subsets with different functions, designated Th1 and Th2, was first described for mouse T cell clones in 1986. The contrasting functions of the two subsets are associated with different cytokine profiles. Thus Th1 cells produce predominately IFN-γ and IL-2, and are involved in cell-mediated responses to bacteria, whilst Th2 cells produce IL-4, IL-5 and IL-13 and provide help for the B cell production of antibodies, such as IgE produced in allergic reactions. There is strong evidence for the existence of similar subsets of CD4⁺ T helper (and CD8⁺ T cytotoxic) cells in humans, but the production of cytokines is, in some cases, less restricted than in mouse T cells.

Previous evidence had indicated that IFN-γ played an important role in the psoriatic process. This was confirmed by polymerase chain reaction (see below) analysis of biopsies of lesional skin, and measurement of cytokines produced by T cell clones isolated from skin lesions. Both approaches clearly showed that psoriasis was dominated by a Th1-type immune response [5,6].

T cell receptor analysis

Antigenic peptides bound to MHC Class II antigen on the surface of an antigen-presenting cell stimulate T cells by binding to the T cell receptor. The genes coding for the components of the T cell receptor were identified during the 1980s. There are five variable components (Vα, Jα, Vβ, Dβ and Jβ) together with additional amino acids inserted at the junctions between pairs of these components, which increases variability. Contributions from each of these variable components are required for the recognition of foreign antigenic peptides by T cells.

This knowledge stimulated the first studies of T cell receptor rearrangements in lymphomas, leukaemias and autoimmune diseases using restriction fragment length polymorphism analysis. This involved the digestion of DNA isolated from T cells, followed by separation of the resulting fragments using an electric charge (electrophoresis), transfer to a membrane and the application of a radioactively labelled specific DNA probe, followed by exposure of the filter to film (Southern analysis). This was gradually replaced by use of the polymerase chain reaction (PCR), which been devised and named in the mid 1980s. This technique had the combined advantages of requiring less DNA, taking a much shorter time

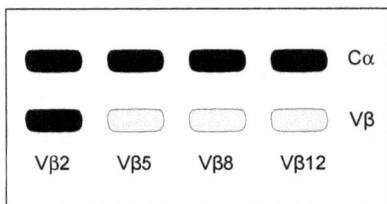

*Representation of an autoradiogram
of TCR transcripts amplified by PCR.
TCR Vβ2 alone is expanded.
(Cα, a conserved chain, is used as a
control in each reaction).*

to perform and not requiring the use of radioactive compounds, making it a safer procedure. At the same time, the range of monoclonal antibodies specific for T cell receptor Vβ families was being expanded. Later, subtypes of several of the Vβ families were recognised, and antibodies to these subfamilies also became available, but antibodies to the Vα families proved more difficult to produce.

Streptococcal superantigens

At the end of the previous decade, a new type of antigen termed "superantigen" was recognised that stimulated T cells almost exclusively via the Vβ region of the T cell receptor[7]. Superantigens did not bind to those regions on the T cell receptor involved in the binding of foreign antigenic peptides, but bound instead to an exposed face of the Vβ chain. Examples of proteins that can act as superantigens are the enterotoxins produced by *Staphylococcus aureus* (e.g. SEC3) and the streptococcal pyrogenic (also known as erythrogenic or scarlet fever) toxins. Each toxin stimulates T cells bearing particular Vβ families that vary for each toxin. In this way a single toxin activates a much larger number of T cells, than does an individual antigenic peptide. This potent T cell

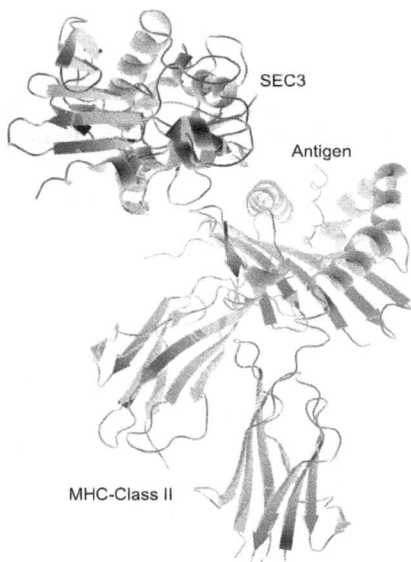

SEC3 complexed with MHC Class II

stimulating activity is probably the major mechanism that bacterial toxins use to cause disease.

The association between streptococcal infections and psoriasis, which had been recognised approximately 40 years earlier, raised the possibility that streptococcal superantigens could play a role in psoriasis. In 1993, this prompted a study of T cell receptor Vβ expression in skin lesions of psoriasis using monoclonal antibodies specific for nine T cell receptor Vβ families[8]. This revealed a marked overexpression of one particular Vβ family (Vβ2) in skin lesions from both guttate and chronic plaque psoriasis patients. A subsequent study by a second research group confirmed this finding in guttate patients and, in addition, showed that the T cells expressing Vβ2 represented many clones capable of recognising a variety of different antigens, suggesting that a superantigen was responsible for their expansion[9]. In support of this, the streptococci isolated from the throats of these guttate patients secreted a toxin called streptococcal pyrogenic exotoxin-C (SPE-C), a superantigen known to stimulate T cells expressing Vβ2.

Disease-associated antigen(s)

The T cell receptor repertoire in chronic plaque psoriasis was analysed in several studies using PCR and DNA sequencing techniques. Preferential usage of particular Vβ families by dermal CD4[+] T cells and epidermal CD8[+] T cells were reported[10,11]. In contrast to guttate lesions, this increased expression was usually associated with a small number of dominant clones (oligoclonality) infiltrating the skin lesions, suggesting expansion *in situ* in response to an antigen or antigens in the skin. Although there was some disagreement between studies as to which Vβ families were preferentially expanded in lesional skin, there was similarity between the reported sequences involved in antigen binding, suggesting recognition of a common disease-associated antigen(s). The identity of this antigen was, and still is, unknown.

Thus the findings of the T cell receptor analysis studies were consistent with a pathogenic role for streptococcal infections in guttate psoriasis, mediated by superantigens. There was also the possibility that other streptococcal products could act as T cell stimulators in the chronic form of the disease, which was also being investigated at this time.

T cell recognition of streptococcal antigens

T cells that proliferated in response to a mixture of streptococcal antigens were cultured from the lesional skin of both guttate and chronic plaque psoriasis patients[12,13]. Although such T cells were also present in other inflammatory skin diseases, they were less frequently isolated, presumably due to their lower numbers. Of significance, however, was the finding that a subset of psoriatic skin T cells produced IFN-γ in response to streptococcal cell wall antigens[14]. In contrast, skin T cells from non-psoriatic inflammatory skin diseases did not show this Th1-type response to streptococcal cell wall antigens. This suggested that the psoriatic Th1 cell response to streptococcal cell wall antigens may be specific for the disease, and therefore of pathogenic significance.

Genetics of psoriasis

It had been recognised as early as the 19th century that psoriasis was an inherited disease, with the first analysis of the genetic basis of this inheritance carried out in 1931 (see Chapter 4). However, it was not until the establishment of the Human Genome Project during the first half of the 1990s that it became feasible to begin a systematic search for the genes determining psoriasis. In 1996, a gene map of the human genome containing 16,000 of the 50,000-100,000 genes then estimated to be present was published[15]. This significant increase in the number of mapped human genes was made possible by the development of high-throughput mapping and sequencing technologies, and opened the way for the location and identification of genes causing a variety of diseases.

Early genetic studies of psoriasis had focused on the association of HLA alleles with the disease. Stronger HLA associations had been found in patients with an age of onset younger than 40 years, and who showed a higher frequency of affected first-degree relatives, than patients with a later onset whose HLA associations were much weaker. The strongest association observed in psoriasis was that of HLA-Cw6, an allele rarely increased in frequency in patients with other inflammatory diseases. However, only a small proportion (approximately 10%) of HLA-predisposed individuals go on to develop psoriasis, suggesting that inheritance of a particular HLA allele is not sufficient by itself for initiation of the disease. Furthermore, it had proved difficult to demonstrate that the HLA associations observed were due to genetic linkage between psoriasis and the HLA locus. Thus it was generally believed that several additional psoriasis genes, triggered by environmental factors, must be involved in disease susceptibility. Some of these genes were likely to be disease-specific, whilst others, with a disease- modulating role, were likely to be present in other immunological diseases.

The first genome-wide linkage study of psoriasis families was published in 1994, and reported a susceptibility locus on chromosome 17q25 (this and subsequent studies reviewed in Ref 16). Interestingly, none of the families with linkage to chromosome 17q showed any association with Cw6, providing the first evidence for the existence of genetic heterogeneity in

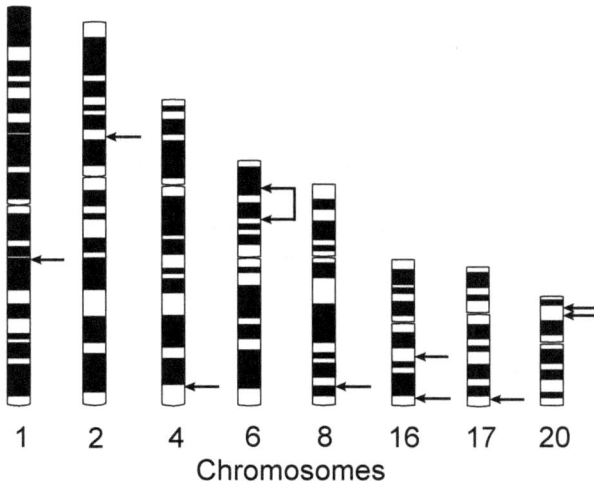

Representation of disease linkage sites in patients with psoriasis, based on data in Ref 16

psoriasis. Two to three years later, susceptibility loci for familial psoriasis were reported on chromosomes 4q 21 and 6p. The susceptibility locus on chromosome 6 was located in the MHC region p21.3, close to HLA-C, as predicted from the HLA association studies. This locus, named PSORS1 (psoriasis susceptibility 1), was subsequently confirmed by several research groups and was found to confer significant risk (35-50%) for development of psoriasis. However, since not all psoriatic patients carry

Cw6, it seemed more likely that the PSORS1 gene was a gene close to HLA-Cw6, rather than Cw6 itself; subsequent studies using more precise mapping methods were consistent with this assumption. Two further candidate genes in this region, coding for corneodesmosin (a glycoprotein expressed in differentiating keratinocytes) and α-helix coiled-coil rod homologue (similar to the hair follicle protein, trichohyalin), have also been investigated. Polymorphisms in both of these genes have been associated with disease susceptibility, but the functional relevance of these genetic changes has yet to be determined.

The identification of 11 further linkage sites on 10 different chromosomes followed during the last few years of the decade[17]. Those loci with statistical evidence of linkage, which had in most cases been replicated, were numbered PSORS2–PSORS7. The rest of the loci showed only suggestive evidence of linkage, although this was, in some cases, replicated in more than one study suggesting that they may represent loci with minor effects.

Candidate genes located at these linkage sites code for proteins involved in epidermal differentiation, immune and inflammatory responses, and response to pathogens, consistent with the current understanding of psoriasis pathogenesis. However, as the millennium came to a close, none of the psoriasis genes had been identified, and HLA-Cw6 had been excluded as the major susceptibility gene for psoriasis.

Laser Treatments

The earliest changes observed in the development of a psoriatic lesion are in the dermal papillary blood vessels, first noted during the 19th century. There is increased proliferation of vascular cells and tortuosity of capillaries, swelling of endothelial cells and widening of the gaps between endothelial cells. It was hypothesised that selective targeting of the cutaneous blood vessels using photothermolysis would block the psoriasis process, allowing resolution of skin lesions. Lesional skin was treated with the flashlamp-pumped pulsed dye laser, the safety of which had previously been established in the treatment of port wine stains. The laser delivered yellow light (585 nm) selectively to superficial blood capillaries at a depth of >1mm, which became heated and thus destroyed. Response rates of between 57% and 82% were reported in treated psoriasis patients, with normalisation of histological features and remission times of up to 15 months.

Excimer lasers were first used as a form of phototherapy in psoriasis in the late 1990s. Excimer lasers operate in the UV range and use a mixture of a noble gas and a halogen, which are induced to form unstable "excited dimers" (excimer) by high energy electric current. The high-energy dimers quickly dissociate to their ground states giving off laser light, which is delivered to its target via a fibre optic cable. These lasers could precisely ablate the surface of a variety of tissues without an apparent thermal effect, termed "cold ablation", but were used only briefly for resurfacing of the skin as they were found to be unsuitable due to technical reasons. The first use of a 308-nm xenon chloride excimer laser as a form of phototherapy in psoriasis was in 1997[18]. Clearance of psoriatic plaques was achieved in 7 to 11 treatments with the laser compared to over 30 treatments with conventional narrow band UVB therapy. In addition to the faster therapeutic effect, the use of the excimer laser has several other advantages, including the sparing of surrounding normal skin from unnecessary UV exposure, long remission times (up to 2 years), and a smaller total cumulative dose needed to clear psoriasis than in conventional phototherapy, thus reducing the potential long-term risk of carcinogenicity from UV exposure.

Topical ascomycins and retinoids

Ascomycin derivatives, a novel class of anti-inflammatory macrolactams, were first introduced in the late 1990s for the treatment of skin diseases. In common with cyclosporin and tacrolimus, ascomycins act by inhibiting cytokine production by T cells, but had the advantage over those two drugs of being effective when applied topically. The main ascomycin compound tested, pimecrolimus, was shown to be effective not only in atopic dermatitis and allergic contact dermatitis, but also in psoriasis under semi-occlusive conditions[19]. It proved to be as effective as topical corticosteroids in these diseases, but had a better safety profile and did not induce skin atrophy.

Retinoic acid was first used to treat psoriasis in the 1970s. Second-generation retinoids, etretinate and its active metabolite acitretin, became part of the psoriasis armamentarium during the 1980s, most commonly combined with UVB or PUVA, but highly effective as a monotherapy for pustular psoriasis. However, they were only administered to patients with severe and recalcitrant forms of psoriasis, because of their attendant toxic side-effects. These side-effects were thought to arise from the non-specific interaction of etretinate and acitretin with several retinoic acid receptors in the skin. The receptors could be subdivided into two families, retinoic acid receptors (RARs) and retinoic X receptors (RXRs). It was therefore hypothesised that if receptor selectivity could be achieved, this would improve the therapeutic profile of the drugs. This led, in the 1990s, to the development of a new class of retinoids called acetylene retinoids, the first of which were tazarotene and tazarotenic acid, which were designed to be selective for RARs. Tazarotene was developed in a topical gel formulation, providing the first topical retinoid for use in psoriasis. Unlike the oral retinoids, the gel was well-tolerated, showed low systemic absorption and was not harmful to foetal development. Furthermore, its beneficial effects in psoriasis were rapid and sustainable over several weeks. Although retinoids were originally believed to act primarily on epidermal cell growth and differentiation, it became evident that their immunomodulatory and anti-inflammatory properties also contributed to the resolution of psoriatic skin lesions.

Biological Therapies

The considerable progress made in determining the role of the immune system in the pathogenesis of psoriasis during this decade, combined with advances in genetic engineering, led to the development of a new class of immuno-modulating biological agents for use in psoriasis[20]. These agents differed from conventional treatments in that, instead of being broadly immunosuppressive, they targeted specific steps in the immune cell pathway leading to psoriasis. In this way, damage to the immune system could be limited, preventing some of the side effects associated with traditional treatments.

Three types of biological agents have been tested in psoriasis; monoclonal antibodies, fusion proteins, and recombinant cytokines. The latter were produced by cloning human cytokine genes into a bacterial genome, allowing the proteins to be produced in large quantities, a technique first introduced in 1973. Monoclonal antibodies, up until this time, had been predominately mouse in origin, which had the disadvantage of inducing neutralising antibodies when used therapeutically. Genetic engineering advances allowed new types of monoclonal antibodies to become available for therapeutic use. These were either chimeric (fused mouse and human sequences, designated "-ximab"), humanized (human backbone with intermittent mouse sequences, designated "-zumab"), monkey sequences (primatized) or fully human. Fusion proteins, on the other hand, were totally human constructs, often between the constant (Fc) portion of an immunoglobulin molecule and the binding site of a receptor (designated "-cept").

These agents were targeted at T cells (or the antigen-presenting cells they interact with) with the aim of blocking T cell activation and proliferation, or were used to inhibit specific cytokines.

As mentioned above, the fusion protein denileukin diftitox and monoclonal antibodies to CD4 were the first examples of the use of biological agents in psoriasis. The diphtheria toxin fusion protein was, however, too toxic for routine use as a treatment for psoriasis. Furthermore, the monoclonal antibodies against CD4 used initially were mouse proteins, which induced the production of human anti-mouse antibodies. This compromised the effectiveness of the therapeutic antibody, allowing only short-term use.

In contrast, the new genetically engineered antibodies were less antigenic, and more compatible with the human immune system. The first of these to be used to treat psoriasis was efalizumab (Raptiva), an antibody raised against the LFA-1 (leukocyte-function-associated antigen-1) molecule expressed on the surface of T cells. Binding of efalizumab to LFA-1 blocks T cell interaction with other cell types, preventing T cell activation and migration through the skin. At the same time alefacept (Amevive), a fusion protein consisting of LFA-3 linked to human IgG, was developed and tested in psoriasis patients. The structure of the fusion protein was designed so that it bound specifically to the target molecule, CD2, expressed by T cells, and was soluble in plasma. The binding of alefacept via its LFA-3 domain to CD2 prevents T cell activation by blocking its interaction with LFA-3 on antigen-presenting cells, and results in the death of the cell. The majority of patients treated with the drug show improvement and remissions can be prolonged, but total clearing is observed in only a small proportion of patients. In addition, several other monoclonal antibodies and/or fusion proteins that block molecules involved in T cell activation or inhibit T cell proliferation were undergoing Phase I or Phase 2 clinical trials in psoriatic patients with varying amounts of success.

The other main targets for these new biological agents are the cytokines released as a result of T cell activation. These mediators play an important role in the psoriatic process by exerting their effects on various cell types in psoriatic skin. The focus of this strategy is the cytokine TNF-α (Tumour Necrosis Factor-α), both because of its increased levels in lesional skin, and the demonstrated efficacy of anti-TNF-α agents such as the fusion protein etanercept (Enbrel) and monoclonal antibody infliximab (Remicade) in RA and/or Crohn's disease. Etanercept and infliximab have the same mechanism of action; they bind to and inactivate TNF-α, preventing the cytokine from binding to receptors expressed on the surface of most types of cell. Both TNF-α inhibitors have been shown to be effective in psoriasis and psoriatic arthritis.

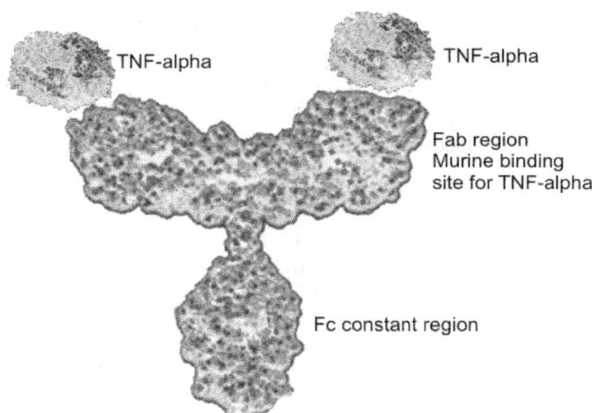

Adapted from: Knight DM, et al. Mol Immunol 1993; 30(16): 1443-53

Infliximab (Remicade) binding to TNF-α

Monoclonal antibodies against other cytokines present in increased levels in skin lesions such as IFN-γ, IL-8 and the subunit shared by IL-12 and IL-23 are also being developed and tested in psoriatic patients, with variable success.

Another approach being employed is that of "immune deviation", which involves the administration of Th2 type cytokines (IL-4, IL-10, IL-11) with the aim of downregulating Th1 cytokine production and/or skewing Th1 cells to a Th2 phenotype. Clinical trials using these recombinant cytokines have demonstrated reductions in Th1 cytokines associated with disease improvement, as predicted, but therapeutic activity is less than that of other immunosuppressive agents.

The development of biological therapies has heralded a new era in the treatment of psoriasis. They have proved both effective and relatively safe in the short to intermediate term; however, it is not known whether there may be side effects associated with long-term use. Furthermore, the high cost of the treatments may be prohibitive, especially in the UK where new drugs have to compete for NHS funding.

Psoriasis in literature
and the media

In addition to extensive coverage in the medical literature over the last century, psoriasis has also been a subject of non-medical literature, both in novels and autobiographies[1].Two authors in particular have published their experiences of the disease and its treatment, and its effect on their lives; the British playwright and novelist Dennis Potter, and the American novelist, John Updike. The Russian novelist, Vladamir Nabokov also suffered from psoriasis, but was more reticent in his writings, preferring not to mention the disease by name.

Dennis Potter

Dennis Potter was born in 1935 to a working class family (his father was a coal-miner) in Berry Hill in the Forest of Dean. He won a scholarship to Oxford University in the 1950s and started writing in 1961 after experiencing a severe bout of psoriasis accompanied by the onset of psoriatic arthropathy. Being bedridden, with a wife and young children to support, Potter wrote his first play for television, *The Confidence Course*. This was accepted by the BBC, who then commissioned him to write another one. This was the start of a prolific writing career, which included 29 plays and 5 each of mini-series, serialized adaptations, novels and films.

His debilitating psoriasis and arthritis laid him up for 6 or 7 months of the year and undoubtedly affected his outlook on life. His work was controversial and sometimes shocking. Indeed, *Brimstone and Treacle*, filmed in 1976, was described as diabolical, even by the author himself. The BBC banned the film for 11 years, and its story of the rape of a physically and mentally handicapped young girl by a handsome young visitor to the family home, provoked much criticism. As his hands became crippled with arthritis, Potter had to strap the pen to his hand as it became difficult for him to write. In the mid 1970s he began taking an anti-cancer drug, Razoxane, which relieved his joint pains and allowed him to work faster. During the next 6 years he wrote probably his best works, including *Pennies from Heaven* and *The Singing Detective*.

The Singing Detective was widely recognised as being autobiographical[2].

Its main character Philip Marlow, a writer of detective stories, is hospitalised with a severe bout of psoriasis and arthritis and relives scenes from his childhood during the 1930s using songs from the past (a characteristic feature of Potter's work) as hallucinations. It was written soon after one of Potter's worse flare-ups in which his entire body was covered in psoriasis, his temperature raised, resulting in hallucinations, and his joints so stiff and painful that he couldn't move. The story is a clear reflection of how he felt about himself at that time.

Potter was less well known in the U.S. as his plays and serializations were less widely broadcasted than in Britain. Furthermore when *Pennies from Heaven* was adapted from the original BBC mini-series by Potter into a film starring Steve Martin in 1981, it did not receive good reviews in the U.S. In the early 1990s, Potter wrote a screenplay of *The Singing Detective*, setting it in the U.S. in the 1950s. It was finally brought to the screen by Mel Gibson in 2003 as an independent film, starring Robert Downey Jr as Dan Dark the central character and directed by Keith Gordon, who was careful to abide by the script and Potter's visualisation of the spirit of the work. The National Psoriasis Foundation of the U.S. was also involved in the production of the film providing all the necessary information about the disease[3]. The film gives a very graphic portrayal of psoriasis and psoriatic arthritis (although the word psoriasis is not actually mentioned) and explores the psychological aspects of the disease. The extensive media coverage of the production has raised awareness of psoriasis, both of the physical and emotional aspects. Indeed, some patients regard *The Singing Detective* as an important source of information[4] and certain doctors even recommend it as such.

Tragically the drug Razoxane, which helped Potter to progress with his writing, was subsequently discovered to be carcinogenic. Potter developed pancreatic cancer in 1994, dying 4 months after diagnosis and only weeks after the death of his wife of 35 years of breast cancer.

John Updike

John Updike was born in 1932 in Reading, Pennsylvania, the only child of Wesley, a science teacher and Linda, an aspiring writer. During a lonely childhood overshadowed by psoriasis and stammering, he read a great deal and started to write material for school plays and shows, encouraged by his mother. He won a scholarship to Harvard in 1950, graduating with a degree in English in 1954, when he joined The New Yorker as a regular contributor. His first novel was published in 1959. Since then Updike has published numerous novels, more than a dozen short story collections, as well as poetry, literary criticism and children's books.

Aspects of Updike's personal life including his childhood, family, stammer and psoriasis, have often been included as themes in his work. For example, *The Centaur*, a novel published in 1963, and which received the National Book Award in the following year, describes the relationship between a schoolteacher George Caldwell and his son, Peter during the 1940s, with the added dimension that the story is interwoven with characters from Greek mythology[5]. The character of Peter is modelled on Updike himself; both have a schoolteacher father and suffer from psoriasis. In the book, Peter describes the skin lesions on his belly "as if pecked by a great bird, dotted with red scabs the size of coins". He felt humiliated by his condition, hiding his spots in the school locker room, and regarded it as a curse from God intended to make him into a man. Yet at the same time, the texture of the skin lesions also gave him pleasure: "the delight of feeling a large flake yield and part from the body under the insistence of a fingernail must be experienced to be forgiven". In the book, Peter blames his mother for passing on the disease to him, believing that only females could transmit psoriasis to their children. (Updike probably made this wrong assumption because he had inherited psoriasis from his mother, whose mother in turn had also suffered from it).

In addition to *The Centaur,* Updike also wrote another story that focuses on a character, in this case a potter, with extensive psoriasis. From *the Journal of a Leper* (the title a reference to the misdiagnosis of psoriasis as leprosy initiated in Biblical times) is written as a diary that describes the experience of the potter as he undergoes treatment with PUVA and his skin lesions resolve[6]. The story focuses on the effect that the clearing of his skin lesions has on his relationship with his mistress, Carlotta. As his skin improves, Carlotta becomes less attracted to him, and him to her (and women in general); furthermore, he loses his artistic flair as a potter. This association between psoriasis and creative ability was also referred to in Updike's memoirs entitled *Self-consciousness* written in 1989, in which he devotes a whole chapter entitled "At war with my skin" to his experience of living with psoriasis[7]. His first psoriatic skin lesions appeared after an attack of measles when he was 6 years old. Treatment consisted of the application of coal tar-containing "siroil", which had little effect apart from softening the scales and whose colour and smell contributed to his embarrassment about his skin, accompanied by abstinence from chocolate and fatty foods. Although the latter produced little visible effect, Updike believed at the time that his skin would have been worse without it. The arrival of summer, with hours spent on the beach exposed to the sun, heralded a temporary retreat of his skin lesions, which reappeared with monotonous regularity during the winter months. He mentions that women were not put off by his skin, but that his war with his skin "had to do with self-love, with finding myself acceptable, whether others did or did not".

However, intensive sun exposure did not come without a price; several incidences of sunburn took its toll on his skin. Eventually at the age of 42 years, sun exposure was no longer effective, and Updike's skin rebelled. Subsequent PUVA treatment, which had just been introduced at Massachusetts General Hospital, Boston during the late 1970s, cleared his skin, but after several episodes of deep burns, he was forced to discontinue the treatment. He was subsequently treated with the drugs methotrexate and etretinate.

Vladamir Nabokov

Vladamir Nabokov was born in 1899 into an old noble Russian family of considerable wealth. The Russian revolution forced him to flee Russia for Europe, and subsequently, when France was occupied by Hitler, to emigrate to the USA. By the late 1930s, Nabokov and his wife were living in poverty, supported only by his income from writing. It was not until the success of his novel *Lolita* at the age of 60 years that he became wealthy again.

Unlike Potter and Updike, Nabokov was reticent about writing or talking about his experience of psoriasis, not even mentioning the term during interviews conducted in the 1970s. However, his biographer, Brian Boyd documented how, in 1937, the nervous tension associated with hiding an illicit love affair with another woman from his wife, precipitated a severe attack of psoriasis that drove him to the brink of suicide[8]. He later wrote to his wife Véra that "I've put on weight, got a tan, changed my skin", referring to the improvement that sunbathing and free radiation treatments from a Russian physician had made to his psoriasis.

Nabokov devoted only one page of his novel *Ada* published in 1969 to psoriasis, again without mentioning it by name[9]. It was mentioned as a "spectacular skin disease that has been portrayed recently by a famous American novelist in his Chiron and described in side-splitting style by a co-sufferer who wrote essays for a London weekly". It is not clear who the latter was, but the American novelist was undoubtedly John Updike. In the book, two individuals with the "spectacular skin disease" recommend treatments to each other, whilst other advice is quoted from an encyclopaedia, which involves taking warm baths at least twice a month and avoiding spices. A reference is also made to the confusion of psoriatic with lepers in the Middle Ages. When he had finished writing this book in the late 1960s, Nabokov suffered a flare-up of his psoriasis, which was the only other mention of his skin condition made by his biographer.

Other authors, such as Kazuo Ishiguro, have also included the subject of psoriasis in their novels. Ishiguro features a character called Leo Brodsky with the disease in a book entitled *The Unconsoled*, but, in common with Nabokov, psoriasis was not mentioned by name by the author.

~ 12 ~

The 21ˢᵗ Century and the Future

Two hundred years after it was first recognised as a distinct clinical entity, psoriasis has now been firmly established as a polygenic disease, triggered by environmental factors and mediated by T cells, and with a possible autoimmune component.

In the coming years, it is likely that both the genes that determine susceptibility to psoriasis, and the bacterial antigen(s)/autoantigen(s) that trigger or maintain the disease process will be identified. This increase in our understanding of the aetiology of psoriasis will, in turn, allow the development of novel therapies that more specifically target the disease pathway, with the ultimate aim of switching off the disease permanently.

Changing theories during 200 years of psoriasis

It was generally believed at the beginning of the 19ᵗʰ century that psoriasis was the result of an internal metabolic disturbance requiring the traditional methods of treatment, such as bleeding and purging . This view gradually changed as the century progressed, when characteristics of the natural history of the disease and the histology of skin lesions became known, and it was recognised that psoriasis was inherited in families (Table). The idea that the defect in psoriasis originated in the epidermis was first proposed in 1930, and during the 1960s, research was focused on the mechanisms underlying abnormal epidermal proliferation in skin lesions. This led to the hypothesis that psoriasis was caused by altered regulation of epidermal cell growth in response to unknown stimuli. In the following decade, autoantibodies to skin antigens were discovered in psoriatic patients. Although these were not specific for the disease, their presence in the epidermis became the basis for further pathogenesis theories, which were later discarded. During the same period, a defective cAMP cascade was proposed as the basis for the development of psoriasis, but there was little convincing evidence that a defect of this kind was of a primary nature. During the 1980s and 1990s, T lymphocytes took centre stage, and several different observations provided irrefutable evidence that T cells were responsible for mediating the psoriatic process. It appears unlikely,

Table. Unravelling of the pathogenesis of psoriasis

Time Period	Significant observations and hypotheses
19th ©	Heredity of psoriasis recognised. Role of infections first considered. Histology of skin lesions described.
1900-30	Samberger hypothesis: primary defect located in epidermal cells
1930-39	Definition of psoriatic arthritis. First reports of association with strep infection. First genetic studies of twins and psoriatic pedigrees.
WWII	
1950-59	ASLO antibody titres confirm strep association with guttate psoriasis. First use of tonsillectomy to treat psoriasis. Steinberg hypothesis: Minimum of 2 genes involved in predisposition to psoriasis.
1960-69	Farber & Cox hypothesis: Inherited defective epidermal growth regulation in response to unknown stimuli.
1970-79	HLA associations investigated - proposed linkage of Cw6 to a psoriasis gene. Autoantibodies observed bound to epidermal cells. Two resulting hypotheses: Beutner - anti-stratum corneum Cormane - anti-basal cell nuclei First studies of skin cellular infiltrate. Voorhees & Duell hypothesis: defective cAMP cascade.

Time Period	Significant observations and hypotheses
1980-89	Monoclonal antibodies used to characterise T and dendritic cells in skin lesions. Valdimarsson hypothesis: Epidermal growth induced by T cell-derived factor. T cell and keratinocyte-derived cytokines identified in skin lesions. First mouse models of psoriasis used to locate defect in the skin
1990-99	Several observations support hypothesis that psoriasis is mediated by T cells. T cells in skin lesions characterised. T cell response to streptococcal antigens/superantigens demonstrated. Search for psoriasis genes initiated – 14 linkage sites on 13 chromosomes identified
21st ©	Ongoing areas of research: Identification of psoriasis genes and their role in the disease. Search for antigens/autoantigens that activate pathogenic T cells Investigation of the innate immune response to pathogens

however, that defects in the immune system are sufficient by themselves to cause the disease without a simultaneous alteration in epidermal cell function. Genetic studies carried out at the end of the 20th century (see below) are consistent with this hypothesis.

T cells, Antigens and Autoantigens

It has been established over the last two decades that psoriasis is a T cell-mediated disease. CD4+ T cells are essential for initiating and maintaining the psoriatic process, and, when removed by treatment, the disease is temporarily switched off. However, less is known about the function of CD8+ T cells in skin lesions. It is now generally believed that CD8+ T cells play an active role in chronic plaque psoriasis, probably via their ability to produce IFN-γ (and probably other cytokines) that contribute to excessive epidermal cell growth. However, since it has not been possible to remove CD8+ T cells from lesional skin without also deleting CD4+ T cells, it is not known how essential they are to the psoriatic process. In contrast in guttate psoriasis, which often resolves spontaneously, the role of CD8+ T cells may be to inhibit rather than assist the function of CD4+ T cells, thus switching off the disease process.

Both dermal CD4+ T cells and epidermal CD8+ T cells each consist of small numbers of dominant clones that have expanded *in situ*, suggesting that antigens drive the disease process. The identity of these antigens is unknown, but research has focused on the possibility that CD4+ T cells may be specific for a bacterial antigen(s). Indeed, a recent study has implicated a major component of the streptococcal cell wall, peptidoglycan, as an activator of CD4+ T cells in psoriasis[1]. Furthermore, macrophages containing bacterial peptidoglycan have been observed close to CD4+ T cells in psoriatic skin lesions. It remains to be established, however, whether these streptococcal peptidoglycan-specific T cells are responsible for causing disease. It is likely that other components derived from yeasts (*Malassezia* and *Candida albicans*) or viruses (HIV, retroviruses, papillomaviruses), which are associated with the triggering and/or exacerbation of psoriasis, may also be T cell activators in some patients.

Peptidoglycan (along with many other conserved molecules expressed by microorganisms) is a strong activator of innate immunity; the immediate, non-specific response to pathogens which precedes the T cell response. Innate immunity in psoriasis has become a current focus of research as evidence is emerging that the response to pathogens is dysregulated, with a marked increase in the production of anti-bacterial peptides.

Psoriasis has long been assumed to be an autoimmune disease, partly because of its HLA associations, infiltration by T cells, and persistence throughout life, but T cells that recognise a self-antigen have yet to be

110

isolated from skin lesions. Some evidence suggests that keratin, present in epidermal cells, could be a possible stimulus for antigen-specific CD8[+] T cells in the epidermis, and that this might result from cross-reactivity caused by a similarity in structure between keratin and the M protein expressed on the cell wall of streptococci[2]. A search for other keratinocyte proteins that could act as psoriasis antigens as a result of their similarity to streptococcal proteins (antigen mimicry) could prove to be a fruitful area of research in the future.

Overall, these findings suggest that psoriasis may be an autoimmune T cell disease, triggered by an infection. Such a hypothesis has been proposed for various other autoimmune diseases such as diabetes and multiple sclerosis.

Genes

Psoriasis is a complex polygenic disease, and after more than 10 years of genetics research, the susceptibility genes involved are still unknown, although candidate genes have been proposed with varying amounts of supporting evidence. A major locus (PSORS1) for psoriasis has been confirmed in the MHC region on chromosome 6p in several independent studies, but the identity of the gene close to HLA-C still remains to be identified. The number of reported genetic linkages to psoriasis has now grown to a staggering 19 loci on 15 different chromosomes. Although some of these may not be confirmed as true linkages, it is clear that several genes are necessary for psoriasis to develop, and that clinical heterogeneity is probably explained by the inheritance of different combinations of genes in different families. Furthermore, some linkage sites for psoriasis appear to overlap with those identified for other inflammatory and autoimmune diseases such as atopic dermatitis, Crohn's disease, RA and SLE[3]. This suggests that there are common mechanisms underlying these immune-based diseases, in addition to the specific defects that determine their organ specificity and presentation.

Candidate genes that have been proposed in psoriasis include those coding for proteins that are involved in differentiation of epidermal cells, immune and inflammatory processes or responses to pathogens. As technology advances further over the next 10 years, it is likely that the identity of the major genes that predispose to the disease will eventually be revealed, allowing a better understanding of why psoriasis develops in certain individuals and what determines how it is expressed.

Treatments

From the perspective of a new century, how much safer and effective are the therapeutic options now available for patients with psoriasis as compared to 100 years ago?

Although treatments improved greatly during the last century, largely because they became evidence-based, patient dissatisfaction was still high, as shown by a large patient survey carried out by the National Psoriasis Foundation in 1998[4]. Traditional treatments for moderate to severe psoriasis, some of which have been in use for several decades (Figure), have many limitations including immunosuppressive effects leading to an increased risk of infection and cancer, toxicity, a requirement for continual monitoring and inconvenience of use. This has contributed to an increasing use by psoriatic patients of over the counter medications, and complementary or alternative forms of medicine. Herbal remedies, nutrition therapy, traditional Chinese remedies, acupuncture or homeopathy are used by around half of psoriatic patients, mainly as a complementary treatment rather than as an alternative to conventional therapies. This suggests a need for research into the complementary therapies that work best in psoriasis, so that the quality of life of patients undergoing conventional treatments can be improved.

The introduction of biological therapies at the end of the 20th century represented a new, more specific approach to the treatment of psoriasis, based upon an increased understanding of the role of the immune system in the pathogenesis of the disease (see Chapter 10). Alefacept, efalizumab, etanercept and infliximab have all now been been approved by the US Food and Drug Administration (FDA), and its European equivalent (EMEA), for use in psoriasis; the latter two are also approved for psoriatic arthritis. Assessments of the performance of these agents in psoriasis over a 3 to 5 year period concluded that they were not only effective, but non-toxic and relatively safe[2,3]. Furthermore, their use required less monitoring, and they were more convenient and easy to administer. Thus biological agents appear to provide a safe and effective alternative to traditional therapies, although long-term safety data is lacking.

Despite these obvious advantages biological therapies, in common with all previous treatments, cannot induce permanent remission of the disease. However, you would be excused from thinking that a cure for psoriasis

Introduction and length of use of main treatments for psoriasis

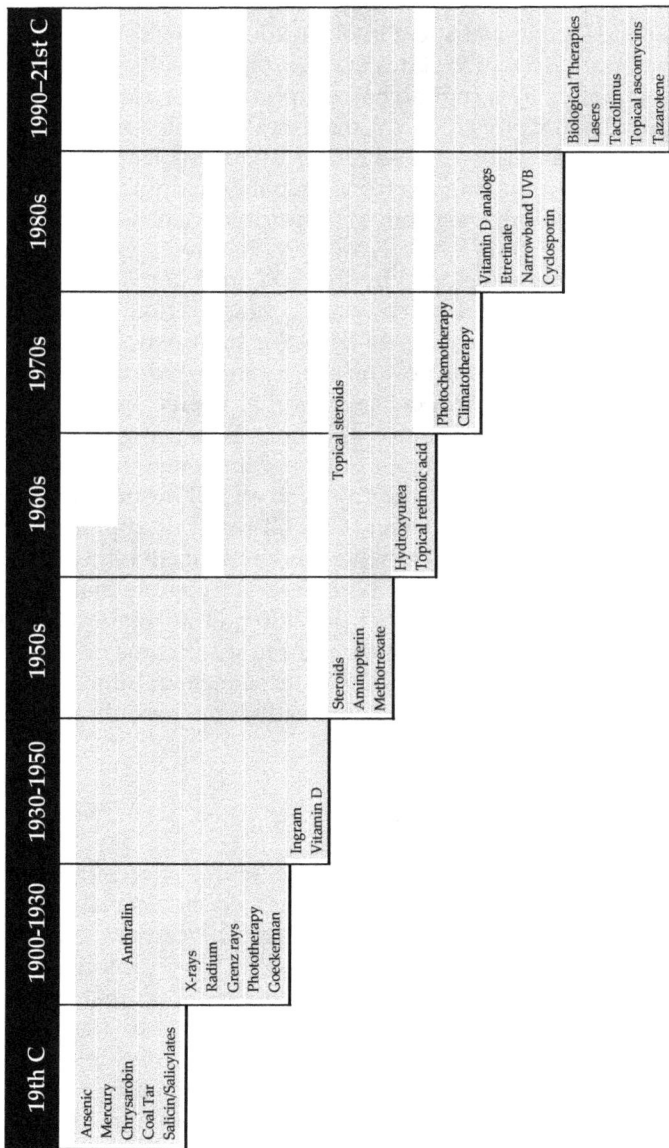

	19th C	1900-1930	1930-1950	1950s	1960s	1970s	1980s	1990–21st C
	Arsenic							
	Mercury							
	Chrysarobin	Anthralin						
	Coal Tar							
	Salicin/Salicylates							
		X-rays						
		Radium						
		Grenz rays						
		Phototherapy						
		Goeckerman						
			Ingram					
			Vitamin D					
				Steroids				
				Aminopterin				
				Methotrexate				
					Hydroxyurea	Topical steroids		
					Topical retinoic acid			
						Photochemotherapy		
						Climatotherapy		
							Vitamin D analogs	
							Etretinate	
							Narrowband UVB	
							Cyclosporin	
								Biological Therapies
								Lasers
								Tacrolimus
								Topical ascomycins
								Tazarotene

113

exists when you "surf the net", as psoriasis patients increasingly do in the search for safe and effective remedies, as the Internet advertises a whole range of treatment regimes for "curing" psoriasis. For example, you could buy from one dedicated website a book entitled "Psoriasis can be cured" by Dr Robert Connolly, which states that psoriasis results from an internal dysfunction treatable by a regime based upon "Bioenergetics", involving self-treatment of neurophysiological areas, herbal tablets and diet. Or, you could choose from a variety of "secret formulas" which claim to banish skin lesions forever, many of which are probably no more than expensive moisturising creams with coal tar or steroids added. Occasionally one of these advertised creams is showcased by the media, such as the anti-bacterial barrier cream developed by Brian Bennett, a retired lorry driver from Nuneaton, to help relieve his wife's contact dermatitis. This cream, used to prevent MRSA infection and in the treatment of various skin diseases including psoriasis, is now on sale in some Asda stores. However, not everyone agrees that it works as well as has been claimed. That is not to say that some patients do not receive benefit from using these creams or following these therapeutic regimes, but it is debatable whether this is due to the cream/regime itself or to the "placebo effect" induced by the belief that it will work. (The placebo effect is a well-recognised phenomenon in which a patient's disease improves when given an inactive substitute in the belief that he/she is receiving the active drug). The commercial sites selling these "miracle cures" on the Internet provide no information about risks or side effects, no list of ingredients present in the creams or any support for their claims of beneficial effects. With these facts in mind, using these preparations could involve some risk to health, or at best, disappointment if there is no improvement of skin lesions.

Future research and treatments

So, is there any chance that a real cure will emerge in the future? Well, just as the biological agents have emerged as a result of a greater knowledge of the role of T cells in psoriasis, so the next generation of drugs will depend upon further insights into the immunopathogenic process. Determination of the nature of the antigen(s) that triggers the disease, the characterisation of pathogenic T cells and the identity of disease susceptibility genes are all in reach during the next few years. This knowledge will enable pathogenic T cells to be targeted specifically, thus reducing the side effects caused by indiscriminate killing of activated T cells in general. One way this could be achieved is by the development of a specific T cell vaccine prepared from an individual patient's own T cells, as has been recently reported for the treatment of multiple sclerosis and SLE[7,8]. The mechanism of action remains to be fully elucidated but appears to involve the induction of a subset of T cells that inhibit the function of pathogenic T cells. Alternatively, identification of the genes that predispose an individual to developing psoriasis may allow the disease to be switched off via gene manipulation. So-called "anti-sense" molecules are already being developed that prevent protein formation by binding to messenger RNA released by an activated gene. Application of such molecules to psoriatic skin could allow modification of defective epidermal genes, thus inhibiting abnormal epidermal cell proliferation. In addition, further progress in the field of pharmacogenetics, the study of how genes determine an individual's response to drugs, will enable new and/or existing treatments to be tailored to individuals, increasing the likelihood of a successful outcome.

Clearly there is much still to be learnt about the processes that result in the formation of psoriasis skin lesions. It is expected that answers to many of the questions now posed will emerge during the 21st century in association with further progress in technological advances. However, the ultimate aim, after 200 years of observation, research and treatment of psoriasis, is to find a cure for this common skin disease.

References

Chapter 1

1. Bryan C.P. The Papyrus Ebers. New York, D.Appleton & Co., 1931.
2. Bechet P.E. Psoriasis; a brief historical review. Arch. Dermatol. 1936; 33: 325-334.
3. Zias J. & Mitchell P. Psoriatic arthritis in a fifth-century Judean Desert monastery. Am. J. Phys. Anthropol. 1996; 101: 491-502.
4. Jopling W.H. & Jones B.E.A. Psoriasis and leprosy. J. Am. Acad. Dermatol. 1990; 22: 321.

Chapter 2

1. Hebra F. On Diseases of the Skin. Vol. 1. Translated by C.Hilton Fagge, 1866
2. Köbner H. Zur Aetiologie Ppsoriasis. Vjschr. Dermatol. 1876; 3: 559.
3. Lang. Archiv. 1878; v: 443.
4. Ries. Archiv. 1888; xv: 871.
5. Rohe G.H. Two cases of acute general psoriasis following vaccination. J. Cutan. Venereol. Diseases 1882; 1(1): 11-15.
6. Jamieson W.A. The Histology of Psoriasis. Edinburgh Med. J. 1879; 24 (7): 622-29.
7. Munro W.J. Note sur l'histopathologie du psoriasis. Ann. Dermatol. Syph. 1898; 9: 961-7.
8. Bulkley L.D. Clinical study and analysis of 1,000 cases of psoriasis. Reprinted from Maryland Med. J., Journal Publishing Co., Baltimore, 1891, pp16.
9. Bulkley L.D. Clinical notes on psoriasis with especial reference to its prognosis and treatment. Reprinted from Transactions Med. Soc. New York, 1995, pp14.
10. Girdlestone T. Observations on the effects of Dr Fowler's mineral solution in lepra and other diseases. Med. Phys. J. London 1806; 15: 298-301.
11. Shapter L. Treatment of psoriasis by arsenic in large doses. Lancet 1878 Oct 5; 112(2875): 474-6.
12. Duckworth D. Clinical notes on the diagnosis and treatment of psoriasis. Lancet 1874 July 4; 104(2653): 7-9 .
13. Bramwell B. Atlas of Clinical Medicine. 3 Vols. Edinburgh: T and A Constable at the University Press, 1896.
14. Crocker Radcliffe H. Salicin and salicylates in the treatment of psoriasis and some other skin affections. Lancet 1895 June 8; 145(3745): 1421-3.
15. McNab J. The Lancet 1870 Mar 19; 95(2429): 408-9.
16. Thin G. The treatment of psoriasis by pyrogallic acid. Lancet 1881 April 9; 117(3006): 576.

Chapter 3

1. Serrell Cooke A.D. A note on psoriasis from a bacteriological point of view. Lancet 1910 Nov 26; 176(4553):1548.
2. Wachowiak M. et al. The occurrence of monilia in relation to psoriasis. Am. Archiv. Dermatol. Syphil. 1929; 19: 713.
3. Strickler A. & Asnis E. Blood studies in psoriasis. Archiv. Dermatol. Syphil. 1923; 8: 521.
4. Winfield J.McF. J.Cut.Dis 1916; 34: 441.
5. Samberger F. Further observations on the nature of psoriasis. Prague Dermat. Woch 1930; xc: 261.
6. MacKee G.M. In: X rays and radium in the treatment of diseases of the skin. 2nd Edition, Henry Kimpton, London, 1927.
7. NY Derm Soc. Meeting. Archiv. Dermatol. Syphil. 1920; 2: 260.
8. Crocker H.R. The therapeutic effect of radium emanations in some diseases of the skin. Lancet 1909 Nov 13; 174(4498): 1447-8.
9. Edwards E.K. & Edwards E.K. Grenz ray therapy. Int. J.Dermatol. 1990; 29: 17-18.

10. Goeckerman W.H. The treatment of psoriasis. Northwest Med. 1925; 24: 229-31.
11. Muller S.A. & Perry H.O. The Goeckerman treatment in psoriasis: Six decades of experience at the Mayo clinic. Cutis 1984; 34: 265-70.
12. Galewsky. Uber Cignolin, ein Ersatzpraparat des Chrysarobins. Dermatol. Wchnschr. 1916; 6: 113-5.
13. Unna P.G. Cignolin als Heilmittel der Psoriasis. Dermatol.Wchnschr. 1916; 6: 116-37, 151-63, 175-83.
14. Chalmers Watson D. & Douglas Thompson J.A. The treatment of psoriasis with myelocene. Lancet 1902 Oct 18; 160(4129): 1033.

Chapter 4

1. Hunt E. Psoriasis and rheumatism. A comparison. Lancet 1933 Aug 12; 222(5737): 351-2.
2. Barber H.W. Psoriasis unconquered. Lancet 1940 Nov 30; 236(6118): 696-7.
3. Benedek T. Rheumatoid arthritis and psoriasis vulgaris: internal and cutaneous manifestations of the permanent endoparasitism in the Homo sapiens, their common aetiology, pathogenesis and specific vaccine therapy. Ann Arbor, 1955.
4. Hoede K. Umwelt und Erblichkeit bei der Entstehung der Schuppenflechte. Wurzb Abh Med 1931; 27: 211-54.
5. Ceder E.T. & Zon L. Publ.Health Rep., Washington. Nov 5, 1937; 1580.
6. Gold S. Undecylinic acid in psoriasis. Lancet 1950 Aug 12; 256(6624): 270- 271.
7. Bos J.H. & Farber E.M. Joseph Stalin's psoriasis: its treatment and the consequences. Cutis 1997; 59: 197-199.

Chapter 5

1. Weyers W. Death of medicine in Nazi Germany: Dermatology under the Swastika. Philadelphia; Ardor Scribendi. 1998.
2. Macpherson W.G., Herringham W.P., Elliott T.R., Balfour A., eds. Medical services. Diseases of the war. In: History of the Great War, Vol 2, London, England. His Majesty's Stationery Office, 1923, p68.
3. Wittkower E. Psychological aspects of psoriasis. Lancet 1946 April 20; 247(6399): 566-569.
4. Simons R.D.G. Additional studies on psoriasis in the tropics and in starvation camps. J. Invest. Dermatol. 1948; 12: 285-294.
5. Zackheim H.S. & Farber E.M. Rapid weight reduction and psoriasis. Arch. Derm. 1971; 103: 136-140.
6. Gans O. Some observations on the pathogenesis of psoriasis. Arch. Dermatol. Syphil. 1952; 66: 598-611.
7. Grütz O. & Bürger M. Die Psoriasis als Stoffwechselproblem. Klin.Woch. 1933; 12: 373.
8. Swartz JH. The possible inter-relation of psoriasis and *Streptococcus faecalis*. N. Engl. J. Med. 1945; 233: 296-7.

Chapter 6

1. Romanus T. Psoriasis from a prognostic and hereditary point of view. Acta Dermatol. Venereol. Stockholm 1945; 26(Suppl 12): 1-137.
2. Steinberg A.G., Becker S.W., Fitzpatrick T.B., Kierland R.R. A genetic and statistical study of psoriasis. Am. J. Hum. Genet. 1951; 3: 267-81.
3. Norrlind R. The significance of infections in the origination of psoriasis. Acta Rheum. Scand. 1954; 1: 135-144.
4. Norholm-Pedersen A. Infections and psoriasis. A preliminary communication. Acta Dermatol. Venereol. 1952; 32: 159-67.
5. Whyte J. & Baughman R.D. Acute guttate psoriasis and streptococcal infection. Arch. Dermatol. 1964; 89: 350-356.
6. Wright V. Rheumatism and psoriasis. A re-evaluation. Ann. J. Med. 1959; 27: 454-62.
7. Lodge E. Triamcinolone in chronic psoriasis. Lancet 1959 24 Jan; 273(7065): 186-7.
8. Gubner R., August S., Gincberg V. Therapeutic suppression of tissue reactivity. II. Effects of aminopterin in rheumatoid arthritis and psoriasis. Am. J. Med. Sci. 1951; 221: 176-82.

9. Gubner R. Effect of "aminopterin" on epithelial tissues. Arch. Dermatol. Syphilol. 1951; 64: 688-99.
10. Rees R.B., Bennett J.H., Bostick W.L. Aminopterin for psoriasis. AMA Arch. Dermatol. 1955; 72: 133-144.
11. Edmundson W.F. & Guy W.B. Treatment of psoriasis with folic acid antagonists. AMA Arch. Dermatol. 1958; 78: 200-3.

Chapter 7

1. Van Scott E.J. & Ekel T.M. Kinetics of hyperplasia in psoriasis. Arch. Dermatol. 1963; 88: 373-81.
2. Weinstein G.D. & Van Scott E.J. Autoradiographic analysis of turnover times of normal and psoriatic skin. J. Invest. Dermatol. 1965; 45: 257-62.
3. Goodwin P., Hamilton S., Fry L. The cell cycle in psoriasis. Brit. J. Dermatol. 1974; 90: 517-24.
4. Weinstein G.D. & Frost P. Abnormal cell proliferation in psoriasis, J. Invest. Dermatol. 1968; 50: 254-9.
5. Flaxman B.A. & Chopra D.P. Cell cycle of normal and psoriatic epidermis in vitro. J. Invest. Dermatol. 1972; 59: 33-34.
6. Farber E.M. & Cox A.J. The biology of psoriasis. J. Invest. Dermatol. 1967; 49: 348-57.
7. Fry L. & McMinn R.M.H. The action of chemotherapeutic agents on psoriatic epidermis. Brit.J. Dermatol. 1968; 80: 373-83.
8. Skog E. & Linder O. Immunologic studies in pathologic conditions of the skin, with special reference to psoriasis. Acta Dermatol. Venereol. 1965; 45: 461-466.
9. Ausum J.D. & Wilhelm R.E. Psoriasis (Immunological studies). Arch. Dermatol. 1962; 85: 614-6.
10. Leavell U.W. & Yarbro J.W. Hydroxyurea. A new treatment for psoriasis. Arch. Dermatol. 1970; 102: 144-50.
11. Frost P. & Weinstein G.D. Topical administration of vitamin A for ichthyosiform dermatoses and psoriasis. J.A.M.A. 1969; 207: 1863-8.
12. Lomholt G. Psoriasis:Prevalence, Spontaneous Course and Genetics. G.E.C. Gad, Copenhagen, 1963.
13. Hellgren I. Psoriasis: The Prevalence in Sex, Age and Occupational Groups in Total Populations in Sweden: Morphology, Inheritance and Association with Other Skin and Rheumatic Diseases. Almqvist & Wiksell, Stockholm, 1967.
14. Farber E.M., Bright R.D., Nall M.L. Psoriasis: A questionnaire survey of 2,144 patients. Arch. Dermatol. 1968; 98: 248-59.

Chapter 8

1. Karvonen J. HL-A antigens in psoriasis with special reference to the clinical type, age of onset, exacerbations after respiratory infections and occurrence of arthritis. Ann. Clin. Res. 1975; 7: 301-11.
2. White S.H., Newcomer V.D., Mickey M.R. et al. Disturbance of HL-A antigen frequency in psoriasis. N. Engl. J. Med. 1972; 287: 740-3.
3. Hirata A.A. & Terasaki P.I. Cross-reactions between streptococcal M proteins and human transplantation antigens. Science 1970; 168: 1095-6.
4. Guilhou J.J., Meynadier J., Clot J. New concepts in the pathogenesis of psoriasis. Brit. J. Dermatol 1978; 98: 585-592.
5. Beutner E.H., Binder W.L., Jablonska S., Kumar V. Immunofluorescence findings on stratum corneum antibodies, antigens and their reaction in vitro and in vivo as related to repair and psoriasis. In: Beutner EH (ed), Autoimmunity in Psoriasis. CRC Press, Boca Raton, FL, 1982, pp. 53-80.
6. Cormane R.H., Hunyadi J., Hamerlinck F. The role of lymphoid cells and polymorphonuclear leukocytes in the pathogenesis of psoriasis. J. Dermatol. 1976; 3: 247-59.
7. Clot J., Dardenne M., Brochier J., Andary M., Guilhou J.J. Evaluation of lymphocyte subpopulation and T cell functions in psoriasis. Clin. Immunol. Immunopathol, 1978; 9: 389-97.
8. Stingl G., Wolff K., Diem A., Baumgartner G., Knapp W. In situ identification of lymphoreticular cells in benign and malignant infiltrates by membrane receptor sites. J. Invest. Dermatol. 1977; 69: 231-5.
9. Bjerke J.E., Krogh H.K., Matre R. Characterisation of mononuclear cell infiltrate in psoriatic

lesions. J. Invest. Dermatol. 1978; 71: 340-3.

10. Voorhees J.J. Pathophysiology of psoriasis. Ann. Rev. Med. 1977; 28: 467-73.
11. Voorhees J.J. & Duell E.A. Psoriasis as a possible defect of the adenyl cyclase-cyclic AMP cascade. A defective chalone mechanism? Arch. Dermatol. 1971; 104: 353-358.
12. Kragballe K., Desjarlais L., Voorhees J.J. Leukotrienes B4, C4 and D4 stimulate DNA synthesis in cultured human epidermal keratinocytes. Brit. J. Dermatol. 1985; 113: 43-52.
13. Ellis C.N., Fallon J.D., Heezen J.L., Voorhees J.J. Topical indomethacin exacerbates lesions of psoriasis. J. Invest. Dermatol. 1983; 80: 362.
14. Kragballe K. & Herlin T. Benoxaprofen improves psoriasis: a double-blind study. Arch. Dermatol. 1983; 119: 548-52.
15. Guilhou J.J., Meynadier J., Clot J. New concepts in the pathogenesis of psoriasis. Brit. J. Dermatol. 1978; 98: 585-92.
16. Parrish J.A., Fitzpatrick T.B., Tanenbaum L., Pathak M.A. Photochemotherapy of psoriasis with oral methoxsalen and longwave ultraviolet light. N. Engl. J. Med. 1974; 291: 1207-11.
17. Diffey B. The contribution of medical physics to the devlopment of psoralen photochemotherapy (PUVA) in the UK: a personal reminiscence. Phys. Med. Biol 2006; 51: R229-44.
18. Galen. De Simplicium Medicamentorum Temperamentis ac Facultatibus, XI, 2:10 (Kuhn).
19. Even-Paz Z. & Shani J. The Dead Sea and psoriasis. Historical and geographic background. Int. J. Dermatol. 1989; 28: 1-9.
20. Dostrovsky A., Sagher F., Even-Paz Z. et al. Preliminary report: the therapeutic effect of the hot springs of Zohar (Dead Sea) on some skin diseases. Harefuah 1959; 57: 143-45 (Hebrew).

Chapter 9

1. Kohler G. & Milstein C. Continuous cultures of fused cells secreting antibody to predefined specificity. Nature 1975; 256: 495-7.
2. Bos J.D., Hulsebosch H.J., Krieg S.R., Bakker P.M., Cormane R.H. Immunocompetent cells in psoriasis: in situ immunophenotyping by monoclonal antibodies. Arch. Dermatol. Res. 1983; 275: 181-9.
3. Baker B.S., Swain A.F., Valdimarsson H., Fry L. T-cell subpopulations in the blood and skin of patients with psoriasis. Brit. J. Dermatol. 1984a; 110: 37-44.
4. Baker B.S., Swain A.F., Fry L., Valdimarsson H. Epidermal T lymphocytes and HLA-DR expression in psoriasis. Brit. J. Dermatol. 1984b; 110: 555-564.
5. Valdimarsson H., Baker B.S., Jonsdottir I. Fry L. Psoriasis: a disease of abnormal keratinocyte proliferation induced by T lymphocytes. Immunol. Today 1986; 7: 256-9.
6. Luger T.A., Stadler B.M., Katz S.I., Oppenheim J. Epidermal cell (keratinocyte)-derived thymocyte-activating factor (ETAF). J. Immunol. 1981; 127: 1493-8.
7. Swerlick R.A., Cunningham MW., Hall N.K. Monoclonal antibodies cross-reactive with Group A streptococci and normal and psoriatic human skin. J. Invest. Dermatol. 1986; 87: 367-71.
8. Dalen A.B., Hellgren L., Iversen O.-J. et al. A virus-like particle associated with psoriasis. Acta Pathol.Microbiol. Immunol. Scand. 1983; 91: 221-9.
9. Duvic M., Johnson T.M., Rapini R.P. et al. Acquired immunodeficiency syndrome-associated psoriasis and Reiter's syndrome. Arch. Dermatol. 1987; 123: 1622-32.
10. Bjerke J.R., Livden J.K., Degre M., Matre R. Interferon in suction-blister fluid from psoriatic lesions. Brit.J. Dermatol. 1983; 108: 295-9.
11. Griffiths C.E.M., Voorhees J.J., Nickoloff B.J. Characterisation of intercellular adhesion molecule-1 and HLA-DR expression in normal and inflamed skin: Modulation by recombinant gamma interferon and tumor necrosis factor. J. Am. Acad. Dermatol. 1989; 20: 617-29.
12. Baker B.S., Powles A.V., Valdimarsson H., Fry L. An altered response by psoriatic keratinocytes to gamma interferon. Scand. J. Immunol. 1988; 28: 735-40.
13. Schulze H.-J. & Mahrle G. Effects of interferons (rIFN-alpha 2, rIFN-gamma) on DNA synthesis and HLA-DR expression in psoriasis. Arch. Dermatol. Res. 1986; 278: 416-8.
14. Krueger J.G., Krane J.F., Carter M., Gottlieb A.B. Role of growth factors, cytokines and their receptors in the pathogenesis of psoriasis. J. Invest. Dermatol. 1990; 94: 135S-40S.
15. Krueger G.G., Chambers D.A., Shelby J. Involved and uninvolved skin from psoriatic subjects: are they equally diseased? J. Clin. Invest. 1981; 68: 1548-57.
16. Haftek M., Ortonne J.-P., Staquet M.-J., Viac J., Thivolet J. Normal and psoriatic human skin

grafts on "nude" mice: morphological and immunochemical studies. J. Invest. Dermatol. 1981; 76: 48-52.

17.   Baker B.S., Brent L., Valdimarsson H., Powles A.V., Al-Imara L., Walker M., Fry L. Is epidermal cell proliferation in psoriatic skin grafts on nude mice driven by T-cell derived cytokines? Brit. J. Dermatol. 1992; 126: 105-10.

18.   Briggaman R.A. & Wheeler C.E. Jr. Nude mouse-human skin graft model. III. Studies on generalised psoriasis. J. Invest. Dermatol. 1980; 74: 262.

19.   Saiag P., Coulomb B., Lebreton C., Bell E., Dubertret L. Psoriatic fibroblasts induce hyperproliferation of normal keratinocytes in a skin equivalent model in vitro. Science 1985; 230: 669-672.

20.   Braverman I.M., Sibley J. Role of the microcirculation in the treatment and pathogenesis of psoriasis. J. Invest. Dermatol. 1982; 78: 12-17.

21.   Mueller W. & Hermann B. Cyclosporin A for psoriasis. New Engl. J. Med. 1979; 301: 555.

22.   Griffiths C.E.M., Powles A.V., Leonard J.N., Baker B.S., Fry L., Valdimarsson H. Clearance of psoriasis with low dose cyclosporin. Brit. Med. J. 1986; 293: 792-3.

23.   Ellis C.N., Gorsulowsky D.C., Hamilton E.A. et al. Cyclosporine improves psoriasis in a double-blind study. J. Am. Med. Assoc. 1986; 256: 3110-6.

24.   Van Joost T.H., Heule F., Stolz E. et al. Short term use of cyclosporin A in severe psoriasis. Brit. J. Dermatol. 1986; 114: 615-20.

25.   Baker B.S., Griffiths C.E.M., Lambert S., Powles A.V., Leonard J.N., Valdimarsson H., Fry L. The effects of cyclosporin A on T lymphocyte and dendritic cell sub-populations in psoriasis. Brit. J. Dermatol. 1987; 116: 503-10.

26.   Baker B.S., Swain A.F., Griffiths C.E.M., Leonard J.N., Fry L., Valdimarsson H. Epidermal T lymphocytes and dendritic cells in chronic plaque psoriasis: the effects of PUVA treatment. Clin. Exp. Immunol. 1985; 61: 526-34.

27.   Baker B.S., Swain A.F., Griffiths C.E.M., Leonard J.N., Fry L., Valdimarsson H. The effects of topical treatment with steroids or dithranol on epidermal T lymphocytes and dendritic cells in psoriasis. Scand.J. Immunol. 1985; 22: 471-77.

28.   Kaplan R.P., Russell D.H., Lowe N.J. Etretinate therapy for psoriasis: clinical responses, remission times, epidermal DNA and polyamine responses. J. Am. Acad. Dermatol. 1983; 8: 95-102.

29.   Lowe N.J., Kaplan R.P., Breeding J. Etretinate treatment for psoriasis inhibits epidermal ornithine decarboxylase. J. Am. Acad. Dermatol. 1982; 6: 697-8.

30.   Morimoto S. & Kumahara Y. A patient with psoriasis cured by 1 alpha-hydroxyvitamin D3. Med. J. Osaka Univ. 1985; 35: 51-4.

31.   Green C., Ferguson J., Lakshmipathi T., Johnson B.E. UVB phototherapy; an effective treatment for psoriasis. Brit. J. Dermatol. 1988; 119: 691-6.

Chapter 10

1.   Baker B.S. Psoriasis is a T cell-mediated disease. In Recent Advances in Psoriasis: The Role of the Immune System 2000; Imperial College Press, London, p50-60.

2.   Gottlieb S.L., Gilleaudeau P., Johnson R. et al. Response of psoriasis to a lymphocyte-selective toxin (DAB389IL-2) suggests a primary immune, but not keratinocyte, pathogenic basis. Nat. Med. 1995; 1: 442-7.

3.   Wrone-Smith T. & Nickoloff B.J. Dermal injection of immunocytes induces psoriasis. J. Clin. Invest. 1996; 98: 1878-87.

4.   Nickoloff B.J. & Wrone-Smith T. Injection of pre-psoriatic skin with CD4+ T cells induces psoriasis. Am. J. Pathol. 1999; 155: 145-58.

5.   Uyemura K., Yamamura M., Fivenson D.F., Modlin R.L., Nickoloff B.J. The cytokine network in lesional and lesion-free psoriatic skin is characterised by a T-helper type I cell-mediated response. J. Invest.Dermatol. 1993; 101: 701-5.

6.   Schlaak J.F., Buslau M., Jochum W. et al. T cells involved in psoriasis vulgaris belong to the Th1 subset. J. Invest Dermatol. 1994; 102: 145-9.

7.   Marrack P. & Kappler J. The staphylococcal enterotoxins and their relatives. Science 1990; 248: 705-11.

8.   Lewis H., Baker B.S., Bokth S. et al. Restricted T-cell receptor Vβ gene usage in the skin of patients with guttate and chronic plaque psoriasis. Brit. J. Dermatol. 1993; 129: 514-20.

9.   Leung D.Y.M., Travers J.B., Giorno R. et al. Evidence for a streptococcal superantigen-driven process in acute guttate psoriasis. J. Clin. Invest. 1995; 96: 2106-12.
10. Prinz J.C., Vollmer S., Boehncke W.-H., Menssen A., Laisney I., Trommler P. Selection of conserved TCR VDJ rearrangements in chronic psoriatic plaques indicates a common antigen in psoriasis vulgaris. Eur.J. Immunol. 1999; 29: 3360-8.
11. Chang J.C.C., Smith L.R., Froning K.J. et al. CD8+ T cells in psoriatic skin lesions preferentially use T-cell receptor Vβ3 and/or Vβ13.1 genes. Proc. Natl. Acad. Sci. USA 1994; 91: 9282-6.
12. Baker B.S., Bokth S., Powles A. et al. Group A streptococcal antigen-specific T lymphocytes in guttate psoriatic lesions. Brit. J. Dermatol. 1993; 128: 493-9.
13. Baker B.S., Brown D., Porter W. et al. T lymphocytes reactive for group A streptococcal antigens in chronic plaque psoriatic lesions. Arch. Dermatol. Res.1999; 291: 564-6.
14. Brown D.W., Baker B.S., Ovigne J.-M. et al. Non-M protein on the cell wall and membrane of group A streptococci induces IFN-γ production by dermal CD4+ T cells in psoriasis. Arch. Dermatol. Res. 2001; 293: 165-70.
15. Schuler G.D. et al. A gene map of the human genome. Science 1996; 274: 540-6.
16. Henseler T. Genetics of psoriasis. Arch Dermatol. Res 1998; 290(9): 463-76.
17. Elder J.T., Nair R.P., Henseler T. et al. The genetics of psoriasis 2001. The odyssey continues. Arch Dermatol. 2001; 137: 1447-54.
18. Bónis B, Kemény L Dobozy A. et al. 308nm UVB eximer laser therapy for psoriasis. Lancet 1997; 350: 1522 (Letter).
19. Mrowietz U., Graeber M., Brautigam M. et al. The novel ascomycin derivative SDZ ASM 981 is effective for psoriasis when used topically under occlusion. Brit. J. Dermatol. 1998; 139: 992-6.
20. Sterry W., Barker J., Boehncke W.-H. et al. Biological therapies in the systemic management of psoriasis: International Consensus Conference. Brit. J. Dermatol. 2004; 151 (Suppl 69): 3-17.

Chapter 11

1.   Meulenberg F. The hidden delight of psoriasis. Brit.Med. J. 1997; 315: 1709-11.
2.   Potter D. The singing detective. London: Faber and Faber, 1986.
3.   www.psoriasis.org/news/press/2003/20030924_singdetstatement.php
4.   Lanigan S.W. & Layton A. Level of knowledge and information sources used by patients with psoriasis. Brit. J. Dermatol. 1991; 125: 340-2.
5.   Updike J. The Centaur. London: Andre Deutsch, 1963.
6.   Updike J. From the journal of a leper. In: Problems and other stories. London: Deutsch, 1980:181-97.
7.   Updike J. Self-consciousness-memoirs. London: Deutsch, 1989.
8.   Boyd B. Vladamir Nabokov. The Russian Years. London. Chatto and Windus, 1990.
9.   Nabokov V. Ada or Ardor: a family chronicle. London Penguin Books, 1971.

Chapter 12

1.   Baker B.S., Laman J.D., Powles A. et al. Peptidoglycan and peptidoglycan-specific Th1 cells in psoriatic skin lesions. J. Pathol. 2006; 209: 174-81.
2.   Johnston A., Gudjonsson J.E., Sigmundsdottir H. et al. Peripheral blood T cell responses to keratin peptides that share sequences with streptococcal M proteins are largely restricted to skin-homing CD8+ T cells. Clin. Exp. Immunol. 2004; 138: 83-93.
3.   Bowcock AM. The genetics of psoriasis and autoimmunity. Ann. Rev. Genomics Hum. Genet. 2005; 6: 93-122.
4.   Krueger G., Koo J., Lebwohl M. et al. The impact of psoriasis on quality of life. Results of a 1998 National Psoriasis Foundation patient-membership survey. Arch. Dermatol. 2001; 137: 280-4.
5.   Sterry W., Barker J., Boehncke W.-H. et al. Biological therapies in the systemic management of psoriasis: International Consensus Conference. Brit. J. Dermatol. 2004; 151 (Suppl 69): 3-17.
6.   Rich S.J. & Bello-Quintero C.E. Advancements in the treatment of psoriasis: role of biologic agents. J. Manag. Care Pharm. 2004; 10: 318-25.
7.   Achiron A., Lavie G., Kishner I. et al. T cell vaccination in multiple sclerosis relapsing-remitting nonresponders patients. Clin. Immunol. 2004; 113:155-60.
8.   Li Z.G., Mu R., Dai Z.P., Gao X.M. T cell vaccination in systemic lupus erythematosus with autologous activated T cells. Lupus 2005; 14: 884-9.

www.ingramcontent.com/pod-product-compliance
Lightning Source LLC
Chambersburg PA
CBHW071154200326
41519CB00018B/5229